POSITIVE P

TEENAGERS AND SEXUALITY

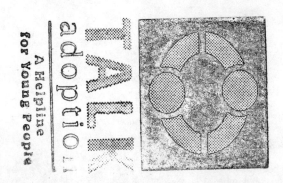

JOHN COLEMAN
OF THE TRUST FOR THE
STUDY OF ADOLESCENCE

Headway · Hodder & Stoughton

British Library Cataloguing in Publication Data

ISBN 0 340 621052

First published 1995
Impression number 10 9   8   7   6   5   4   3   2   1
Year   1999 1998 1997 1996 1995

Typeset by Wearset, Boldon, Tyne and Wear.
Printed in Great Britain for Hodder & Stoughton Educational, a division of Hodder Headline Plc, 338 Euston Road, London NW1 3BH by Cox & Wyman Ltd, Reading, Berks.

Contents

Trust for the Study of Adolescence

The Trust for the Study of Adolescence is an independent research and training organisation based in Brighton. It was established in 1988, and has carried out work in the areas of sexuality, divorce, teenage pregnancy and parenthood, suicide and self-harm, young offenders and adolescent altruism. The Trust has a particular interest in providing support for parents of teenagers. It has published a set of information packs in a series entitled '*Tapes for Parents*'. Each pack consists of a booklet and audiotape of approximately 60 minutes. Titles include:

Teenagers in the Family
Teenagers under Stress
Teenagers and Sexuality
Teenagers and Step-Parents
Teenagers and Drugs
Teenagers and Alcohol

In order to produce these packs Trust staff have interviewed a wide range of parents and teenagers. Some of the interview material from the tapes appears in this book. The Trust may be contacted at 23 New Road, Brighton, East Sussex BN1 1WZ Tel: 01273 693311, Fax: 01273 679907.

Foreword

Change happens so quickly in our society today, that many parents feel out of touch with the world in which their children live. Images of adult sexuality surround them daily, however protective parents may want to be. Some of these images are normal and healthy, others, readily available to most children today, on videos, in magazines, or often on television, need explanation when children come across them. But how as parents can, and do, we explain them all? It's no longer just a matter of coping with simple biological facts – and even those most parents would prefer to be dealt with at school – but increasingly a matter of facing things that we as adults may never have spoken about or understood ourselves.

This is why John Coleman's book is so admirable. Its honest, unembarrassed attitude to every single aspect of teenage sexuality will open the eyes of some parents and give *all* a new insight. It deals so straightforwardly with all those feelings we may prefer to hide. Shame, guilt, anger, and resentment and, above all, embarrassment. Normal feelings in all of us, but who before has offered *us*, the parents, options and a means to cope with this thorny stage of our relationship with the young adults our children are becoming? How to resolve differences of culture, opinion, age and attitude? How to deal with the stresses involved and the sense of failure that overwhelms us all at times?

I suspect that many adults will benefit from this excellent book themselves, finding new ways of talking and behaving that will enhance their own relationships.

In a world riddled with dangers and fraught with ignorance and fear, this book is a breath of fresh air, exemplifying that one thing so often missing from our sexuality – maturity.

Anna Ford

Introduction

This is a book for parents. There are many books, pamphlets, leaflets and so on available for young people, but there are few books which are written for mothers and fathers, step-parents, foster parents and other carers. In the chapters that follow I have attempted to cover some of the issues I believe are of concern to parents. Sexuality is not an easy topic for adults to deal with once their children enter adolescence. Everyone is aware of the need to discuss sex with a teenager. The only question is – how to start the conversation? The experience of this mother and daughter will be familiar to countless parents who have struggled with the problem.

> ❛ And one day I remember I was walking along the track, and Mum said to me "So you know how to do it now then?" So I said well I knew already, you know, because I did. Then she said "You know properly now and all this lot". And I was getting really embarrassed and I was saying yeh, like this, and I was trying to go on to a different subject. And she was saying "So you know how to make a baby and how to look after a baby" and all this rubbish. So I goes "Yes mum" and I was trying to get off the subject all the time. ❜

There is no doubt that the first and overwhelming obstacle is embarrassment. Many people put this down to the poor sex education they themselves received. This may be a factor, but other things play their part. Sexuality causes all sorts of complex feelings within a family, and these feelings have the effect of creating taboos and inhibitions. We will be looking at some of these in the course of this book.

In addition to embarrassment, parents face other difficulties when it comes to dealing with teenage sexuality. Some feel inadequate – uncertain what to say or how to cope with conflicts over values and attitudes. Others find themselves getting anxious about the idea of AIDS, or the possibility of an unwanted pregnancy. Such worries lead them to behave in a fussy or overprotective fashion. On top of all this there are parents who feel quite simply out of their depth. The very idea of talking about sex and sexuality may be something which is quite foreign to them. They realise that their son or daughter is growing up, they know that parents ought to say something, but they are unable to do anything about it.

I hope that all parents, whether shy or anxious, confident or embarrassed, will find something of value in this book.

CHAPTER ONE

Puberty

Puberty is the point in a young person's development when the body begins to change from that of a child to that of an adult. Puberty is not one single event, but many different events, and it takes place over quite a long period of time – usually about two years. Of course sexuality does not begin with puberty. There are many ways in which children make it clear that they are sexual beings. They are curious about their own bodies. They ask questions about their parents' bodies. They may masturbate, or find other ways of giving themselves bodily comfort or pleasure. They are aware of gender differences. All these are reflections of the fact that sexuality develops gradually from infancy onwards. When puberty arrives your child will not be a complete stranger to thoughts and ideas of a sexual nature.

Puberty is, nonetheless, a critical moment in the overall process of growing up. It is during this stage that your child's body develops the characteristics of a sexually mature adult. In addition, a wide range of emotional and psychological changes begin to take place, all of which are part of the essential preparation for adulthood in which every teenager is involved. In this chapter I cover:

- bodily changes in girls
- bodily changes in boys
- the age of puberty
- the emotional consequences of puberty
- periods
- wet dreams.

Bodily changes in girls

The whole process of puberty takes about two years. During this time many different changes occur in the body. For girls the most important of these are:

- the growth spurt (when girls start to grow taller and heavier)
- the development of sexual organs – the uterus, the vagina and so on
- the growth of the heart, the lungs and other major organs of the body
- changes in the composition of the blood and in hormone levels
- the development of the breasts and the hips
- the growth of hair on the body – in particular under the arms and in the pubic area
- the start of menstruation.

When the changes are listed in this way, you can see how puberty affects almost every aspect of bodily functioning. Obviously the changes do not all occur at the same time. For girls the appearance of pubic hair or the beginnings of breast development are most likely to signal the start of puberty. Menstruation is usually something that happens fairly late in the sequence, after hormone levels have altered and internal sexual organs have matured.

Bodily changes in boys

Boys, too, experience many different bodily changes during puberty. The most important of these are:

- the growth spurt (when boys start to grow taller and heavier, and to develop a more muscular body)
- the development of the sexual organs – the penis and the testicles
- changes in the composition of the blood and in hormone levels
- the growth of the lungs, the heart and other major organs of the body
- the breaking of the voice
- the growth of hair on the body – in particular on the face, under the arms and in the pubic region
- the start of wet dreams (when the boy becomes aroused during sleep, and his penis emits semen).

As with girls these changes are very far reaching, and affect all parts of the body. While no two boys progress through puberty in exactly the same way, for most the beginning of the growth spurt indicates the start of puberty, while wet dreams usually occur towards the end of the sequence. Wet dreams indicate that the boy has now become sexually mature.

The age of puberty

Boys and girls differ in the age at which they reach puberty. Boys are usually about 18 months to two years behind girls. On average, in western industrialised countries, girls start puberty between 10 and 11, while boys tend to begin between $11\frac{1}{2}$ and $12\frac{1}{2}$. These figures are, of course, only an average, and it is important to remember that there is enormous individual variation. Imagine a picture of three 13-year-old girls. One is physically still a child, with no breast development, no pubic hair, and no alteration in the shape of the hips. Another is just in the middle of puberty, with the signs of sexual maturity gradually becoming apparent. The third girl is completely mature – she has a woman's body, and is fully developed in all areas. The three girls may at this particular stage feel very different. They look different, their friendships and interests may be different. However in a few years the first two will have caught up with the third, and their differing rates of development will no longer have any significance for them.

There are a few young people – and it is only a small number – who can be classified as late developers. They are two or more years behind the majority in reaching puberty. As far as we know, except in very extreme cases, this has no effect on them as adults. Yet it may make social life difficult for a while. Adults need to be sensitive to the needs of these particular boys or girls. They may well require a bit of extra support or encouragement in making friends or in joining in with others of their own age.

At the opposite end of the spectrum, some children develop earlier than average.

> *Well I think I probably physically changed a lot younger than all of my schoolmates. And that was very embarrassing in a sort of middle school environment. Where, you know, if I was wearing a bra all the boys would go round pinging at me, just being thoroughly annoying. And that was very embarrassing. But with the help of my parents, cos I go home and discuss it with them . . . They'd say you must understand that they're not going through that and they don't know that and so you'll have to bear with it for the moment. After that I think I coped with it very well. But it was very difficult at first.*
> *(16-year-old girl)*

Most boys who develop early seem to be at an advantage, since their strength and athletic skills make them popular with the crowd. For early-developing girls the picture is more mixed. Such girls may be socially successful with older boys, but they may be resented by other girls, and therefore excluded from female activities. Also, their physical maturity may not be matched by their emotional maturity. Girls who reach puberty very early may also need some extra support from adults.

The emotional consequences of puberty

Clearly such major bodily changes cannot occur without there being very important psychological consequences. Your child may be unsettled by the changes to his or her body. He or she may feel odd, or feel different. They may sometimes even find that they don't recognise themselves in the mirror. Increased size, new muscles, a strange body – all this needs time to come to terms with, and may well lead to a period of clumsiness and awkwardness. This, together with the physical changes, can make your teenager extremely self-conscious.

Teenagers experience a range of new feelings as a result of hormonal changes. Some of these may be good feelings, but there will also be more moodiness and depression. Adults should not be surprised if, during this stage, young people appear to be more affected by their emotions than previously. They may well swing sharply from one mood to another. All this is quite normal – part of the process of adjusting to the changes of puberty.

Teenagers during this stage are more prone to doubts and uncertainties about themselves. The changing body leads to a changing sense of self, and may well cause a whole range of anxieties. Some of these will have to do with physical concerns. Am I normal? Is my body the right shape? How can I cure my spots? I wish my hair was a different colour. Am I overweight?

Are my breasts too small? Is my penis big enough? And so on.

> *I remember my daughter saying "I've got these
> lumps, I've got these lumps" you know, and it was
> like "oh well, don't worry, you know, it's breasts
> starting to grow". And then it was "but it hurts", so
> then you find out that that's quite normal and they
> don't always grow at the same rate, and she's
> reassured. I think we went through quite a few
> phases of things not being unexpected but not being
> quite how you might have expected them to be, not
> necessarily all that straightforward and sort of minor
> panics. Usually, I would say "don't worry, I'm sure
> it's perfectly normal", but at the same time you
> know they're bound to worry.*
>
> *(Mother of one daughter and two sons)*

Other worries have more to do with social issues about friends, about dating, about the sort of person the boy or girl is, or is going to become. Again, concerns at this stage are important elements of the process of growing up, and are a necessary part of your teenager changing from a child to an adult.

Periods

Since this is a book for parents rather than for young people, we will not go into great detail about periods, and how they start. There are many useful books for teenagers on this subject, and it is certainly a good idea for every family to have one or two around. You will find some suggestions at the end of the chapter.

What sort of problems do parents face when thinking about their daughter's first period? The most obvious issue has to do with preparation. However determined you are to make sure that your daughter is well prepared, in the event it won't necessarily be easy. You may find it embarrassing to talk about – more embarrassing than either of you expects. Or it may be hard to find the right time. When your daughter is nine years old it may seem too early, but at ten it may be too late. Also it has to be said that some children are more open and curious than others. One girl may be chatty and perfectly relaxed about subjects to do with her body, and may like talking intimately with her mother. Another girl – even in the same family – may be shy and awkward when it comes to talking about personal matters.

Parents should make sure that their daughters are properly prepared and well informed about menstruation. The best time to do this is probably just at the point when puberty is beginning. As we have noted, each girl is different, so there is no general rule about the correct age. Parents need to be aware of their daughter's development, and when the first signs of puberty become obvious (such as changes in the girl's breasts) this is the time to start talking about periods. This is also the time when you need to think about buying the first bra (a training bra).

It is important to remember that a girl may be more worried about or frightened of the idea of periods than she can express. The thought of losing blood can cause all sorts of fears – both rational and irrational. These may be difficult to share with anyone, even in the most caring and supportive family. In our interviews with teenagers this was a theme which recurred time and time again.

> I remember my first fear and hating it so much. I
> thought I really don't want to go through this like, for
> so many years. And I hated that, I really did. I sat
> there and screamed and did just not want it at all. It
> wasn't that I hadn't been prepared for it, I mean, I
> knew it was going to happen and everything. But I
> hadn't really prepared for what I was going to feel,
> the sort of feeling that I've got to go through this
> every month, bla, bla, bla, bla, and my mum just
> sort of said yeh, look on it as a gift rather than you

know, sort of like, torture. But I mean to some extent you sort of think I hate going through this every month.

(15-year-old girl)

However well prepared a girl is, there will always be some anxiety or embarrassment associated with the beginning of menstruation. So it is worthwhile to make sure that your daughter has easy access to a suitable book or leaflet, in addition to talking about menstruation. This means that she can seek information at her own pace and in her own way. She may have practical questions which seem too silly to ask anyone about, or she may be fearful about something which is too embarrassing to acknowledge.

I mean I can remember the first day I learnt about periods from my friend. I was saying oh no, you know, I was terrified. I couldn't believe it and I went home and asked my mum and she told me it was true. And I expected my mum to say no, no it's not true, and I was terrified.

(14-year-old girl)

Not all girls will be living with their own mother. Some may be cared for by fathers, stepmothers, foster mothers or other carers. In such circumstances it may be even more difficult for the teenager to ask difficult questions, or share intimate worries and concerns. It is all the more important, therefore, for carers to ensure that girls know where to go for the information they need.

Finally, it is worth noting that girls today start their periods earlier than they did 10 or 20 years ago. This trend towards early puberty has been going on throughout the twentieth century, and is thought to be the result of better nutrition and healthcare. The practical implications of this are that as many as one in five girls in the last year of primary school in Britain may have started their periods. If your daughter is in this group you need to talk about it with the teachers. You need to ensure:

- that the school has proper facilities for disposing of sanitary towels
- that there is privacy for girls in the toilet area
- that the school has an appropriate sex education policy.

Both boys and girls need to know something about puberty and menstruation in primary school. By the time they reach secondary school it is too late.

Wet dreams

A wet dream happens when a boy becomes sexually aroused during sleep to the point that he ejaculates (his penis emits semen). The first wet dream does not generally have quite the same degree of significance for a boy as the start of periods for a girl. Nonetheless you should not underestimate the importance of wet dreams. Wet dreams can cause a lot of anxiety if the teenager is not properly prepared. The result of a wet dream, such as stains on the sheet, can be acutely embarrassing.

> My youngest son, when he had a wet dream he was terribly embarrassed. Because he was actually going away with my older sons to my sister's for the weekend and I wanted him to take his duvet with him. And he said I can't because it's got lions all over it or something. I said for goodness sake it was Adrian's for five years before it was yours. And I realised he'd had a wet dream all over it, so I had to treat it terribly casually.
>
> *(Mother of three sons)*

Sensitivity on the part of parents or carers is essential. In addition it is obviously important for all boys to be properly prepared. While you don't need to make a big issue of it, simple information,

such as the fact that most boys have wet dreams towards the end
of puberty, will reassure your son.

Conclusion

For the great majority of young people puberty is a natural part of
growing up. Many go through it without thinking very much about
it – it is just something that happens. As one 15-year-old boy said
when asked what he remembered about puberty, 'I hardly noticed
it'. Nonetheless there are some for whom puberty is a worry. This
could be because:

- it comes very early – this may be especially problematic for
  girls
- it comes very late
- it causes anxieties and fears for which the young person is
  not prepared
- the young person is especially self-conscious.

Let me take each of these in turn. First, those girls who start
puberty very early develop breasts and begin their periods before
the rest of their peer group. To be out of step in this way may lead
to embarrassment and awkwardness. It may make friendships with
other girls more difficult. It will certainly mean that boys will pay
extra attention to these girls, making them stand out even more
from the group. Parents, teachers and other adults do need to be
aware of the problems that may arise for these early maturing girls.

Secondly, there will be some, both boys and girls, who reach
puberty much later than the rest. These young people also feel out
of step. They may be excluded from peer group activities, they
may even be bullied. They will probably have all sorts of worries
about the reasons for their late development and what it means for
their future. Consideration, understanding and support from adults
are essential for these teenagers.

Thirdly, there are those who have not been adequately prepared for puberty. Adolescents in this group are not always easy to spot. However, it is worth noting that preparation for puberty is never the responsibility of only one adult. A teacher may be able to provide extra help for a pupil whose family has been disrupted by death or divorce. An aunt or older cousin may be able to offer information to a young person in a situation where the parent is unable to do so. Teenagers should not have to depend on one adult for all the support and information they need.

Lastly, a young person may be particularly self-conscious. This can mean that wearing a bra, or having to undress in a changing room after games, or being shorter than all your friends, causes acute embarrassment. There may not be a lot that adults can do. Nonetheless sensitivity and understanding in the family can make all the difference to a young person whose changing body is causing distress.

For parents, too, puberty may not be much of a problem. Many find issues at this stage easier to deal with than those that present themselves later. However the problems we have just outlined for teenagers can and do lead to difficulties in the home. It is important to recognise, therefore, that puberty is not always easy for parents. Difficulties may arise because of a deterioration in communication or because of marked changes in mood or behaviour. Such changes may seem strange or worrying to parents. However there are likely to be good reasons for the altered behaviour. These are addressed in subsequent chapters of this book, and there are also suggestions for further reading at the end of each chapter.

To conclude, here are the main facts about puberty:

- it is a process that takes place over a period of time
- it involves changes to the whole body, not just to the sexual organs
- there is wide variation between individuals in the timing of puberty
- girls reach puberty earlier than boys

- with puberty comes a whole range of new feelings and emotions
- the changes of puberty can lead to worries and anxieties
- the more information and preparation a young person has, the better.

Useful reading

Have You Started Yet? by Ruth Thomson, Pan Books 1995. This book discusses menstruation, puberty, hygiene and health, including the pros and cons of different sanitary wear. An excellent book for the young teenage girl and her family.

What's Happening To My Body? A Growing Up Guide for Parents and Daughters by Linda Madaras, Penguin 1989. This book covers in detail the physical and emotional upheavals of puberty, with the teenage girl in mind.

What's Happening To My Body? A Growing Up Guide for Parents and Sons by Linda Madaras, Penguin 1989 (revised). A companion book to the above, with excellent information for the teenage boy.

CHAPTER TWO

Learning about sex

It is probably true to say that we learn about sex from the moment of birth. The fact is that the intimacy and nurturing involved in the mother-baby relationship creates a foundation stone for later sexuality. More broadly, however, the child learns about sex from school, from parents, from brothers, sisters, aunts, uncles, cousins and other relatives, from friends and neighbours, from the media, from books and films, from advertising, and from a host of other sources.

As I say I was really young when I first began learning about sex. You sort of pick up words from school and I think I got a rough idea from friends. You see people kissing on TV and you think, well, that must have something to do with it. I didn't really know much about sex at all and then when I saw it in textbooks and stuff like that it became clear. I couldn't say there was ever a time when I just suddenly knew it all, like, when I was twelve. It was sort of a gradual kind of picking it up on the way. Nobody ever sat down and told me. When I heard

my friends talking, I sort of said, oh yea I know that,
you know what I mean? You're dying for them to say
more to see if you can hear more and get a fair idea.
You sort of push them to say more so you pick up
bits like that. It was just a gradual process really that
I learnt about sex. I just didn't sort of like learn it in a
day or whatever.

(17-year-old girl)

Children are curious about sex. After all, it is a fascinating topic. Children are aware of much more that is going on around them than adults realise and, of all the subjects children pay attention to, sex is probably top of the list. When I talk about sex in this context I do not refer specifically to sexual intercourse. Sex is to do with love and relationships, including genitals and their functions, babies and where they come from, differences between men and women, nudity, kissing and physical contact, and much else besides. All these things are part of a large picture, and throughout childhood and adolescence boys and girls are trying to piece together what it all means. Children learn about sex from many different sources, and in this chapter we will be considering the following topics:

- schools
- parents
- society
- friends
- the media
- communication.

Schools

During the 1980s and early 1990s there have been many changes in the legal framework surrounding sex education in schools. Following the Education Reform Act of 1988 the National

Curriculum was introduced into all schools in England and Wales. Unfortunately sex education was not deemed to be part of the National Curriculum, but was defined as a non-compulsory cross-curricular subject. This effectively left it up to individual schools to decide how sex education was to be taught. The onus was placed on school governors to take responsibility for this aspect of the curriculum. As a result there was widespread confusion and uncertainty, and enormous variation between schools in the topics covered and the amount of sex education available to pupils at different ages.

In 1993 a new Education Act came into force in The United Kingdom. This Act placed the biological aspects of sex education within the National Curriculum, and they have therefore become compulsory. Other elements of sex education, particularly those elements to do with relationships, HIV/AIDS and other sexually transmitted diseases, are now deemed to be outside the National Curriculum, however, and the manner in which these topics are taught is left to the discretion of teachers. In addition, parents have been given the right, under the 1993 Act, to withdraw their children from any sex education that does not form part of the statutory National Curriculum. As will be apparent, these changes create a situation which is even more complicated and difficult to understand. Further, the distinction between biological and non-biological aspects of sex education is unclear, and no doubt different schools will come to different conclusions on this issue.

Regrettably, political pressures have been the major factor behind the recent changes in legislation. Since the situation remains unsatisfactory there may well be further alterations in the future. If only politicians, civil servants, church leaders, and media commentators would listen to young people, they would hear a clear and consistent message. Teenagers want more, not less sex education. They want comprehensive and accurate information. They want sex education to come from both the home and the school. Most important of all, they want sex education to cover not only the biological facts of life, but to address the ethical and social issues associated with sexuality. And they want this to be done by someone who can lead an open discussion, rather than by someone who wishes to put across a particular moral viewpoint.

However determined a school is to provide an extensive sex education programme, there are numerous obstacles to be overcome. In the first place, since the mid-1980s there has been an erosion of support for teachers in this area. Local education authorities have been forced to cut back on the numbers of health and sex education advisers, thus reducing the amount of training and assistance available to teachers. Other bodies, such as the Health Education Authority, have had their sphere of operations severely restricted, and in general the current climate within education is not conducive or supportive to the development of high quality sex education. In spite of this there are examples of outstanding work being done in this area. Your child may be lucky enough to attend a school doing such work. Its excellence will almost certainly, however, prove to be the result of individual teachers, and their interest and initiative, rather than of a general sex education policy within the education system.

Another problem faced by teachers is the enormous pressure on curriculum time. As examination results and league tables assume ever greater importance, inevitably non-examination subjects sink to the bottom of the priority list. Perhaps the time has come to rethink these priorities. After all, which is the more important – geography or sexuality? In my view knowing about sexuality is going to have far more of a long-term impact on a child's life than being proficient in geography. What do you think?

A further difficulty for those involved in sex education has to do with values and morality. Indeed much of the political debate has centred around the question of whether sex education should be taught within a 'moral' framework or not. Many argue that sexuality should be taught in the context of ideas about marriage and the family, and often in association with religious beliefs. Others, however, feel that this only alienates young people who may not share the religious views or moral attitudes of their teachers. It is this debate which creates so many of the obstacles preventing schools from providing effective sex education. It should be noted that Britain is not alone here. Similar, possibly worse, problems exist in the USA and in some European countries, such as Italy and Spain. Yet Holland, Sweden and Denmark have managed to pioneer open and worthwhile programmes, and we have much to learn from these countries.

Families from minority ethnic cultures face particular problems here. They may find that their beliefs about sexuality are very different from those of the dominant culture. This can cause conflict, and lead to difficulties between parents, school governors and education authorities. Just as in religious education there needs to be recognition of the many different faiths currently existing in Britain, so in sex education it is essential for schools to acknowledge that there will be different views about sex. Teenagers who are Asian, or Afrocaribbean, or from countries such as Sudan or Cyprus, may find themselves caught between the values of their friends and those of their family. Schools have a critical role to play here in allowing young people to explore these differences. In addition, in the best of circumstances, schools can also help parents from all cultures to learn more about teenagers and sexuality.

Parents

It is very easy for parents to persuade themselves that their child's school is dealing with the tricky and embarrassing issue of sex education. This may let them off the hook, but, as I have just indicated, schools vary enormously in what they do provide. Parents should not take refuge in the comforting thought that 'someone else is doing it'. Parents have responsibilities in relation to sex education. Indeed in the best circumstances the school and the home should work in partnership, each providing different elements of education for sexuality in the widest sense.

> *I like sex education to start at school initially. We've been fortunate in that it has done really for all of my family. I like that because it starts them asking questions and then it's easier for you to go on from that. My own experience as a child was that my parents thought they'd taught me everything and taught me nothing at all. So I had a very confused idea about the whole thing. And my children are all much clearer in the head, even my twelve-year-old knows about how periods are. I mean she has anxiety about it but she has at least got some concept of that and also sexual relationships. I don't suppose she understands the emotional side of it yet, but she again has some idea at least which is much easier to build on. That came from the school really.*
>
> *(Mother of three daughters)*

As far as the school is concerned parents' responsibilities fall into three main areas. In the first place it is up to parents to find out what is being taught. Parents need to know which subjects are being covered, and at what ages. Perhaps most important, they need to know what their son or daughter thinks of the material. Did their teenager still have unanswered questions? Were some topics avoided, or presented too briefly? Were there things the young person disagreed with? And so on. It is true that legislation now requires parents in England and Wales to consent to their children participating in sex education classes. However, this may not necessarily involve the school in providing the family with any great detail regarding the content of the sex education curriculum.

Parents need to know what is going on in school:

- so that they can pick up on issues that are not covered
- so that they can expand on things that are not clear

- so that they can use the school's material as a springboard for open discussion in the home.

There is another reason for parents to keep in close touch with what is taught in school. Research shows clearly that the more interest and concern parents show in schoolwork, the better the young person's performance. Children and adolescents are very sensitive indeed to the way in which their parents value what they do. If parents take school seriously, and demonstrate this by asking questions and wanting to be informed, two messages come across clearly:

- 'I consider this to be important.'
- 'I am interested in you, and in what you are doing.'

Lastly it is worth noting that there are aspects of sexuality which the school simply cannot cover. Sex education in school is likely to be factual, covering reproduction, contraception, sexually transmitted diseases, and so on. Yet we know from research that young people want opportunities to discuss the more personal aspects of sex – the tricky dilemmas of managing relationships and making choices about how to behave. If possible this is better dealt with at home. In addition, with so many pupils in secondary schools it is difficult for teachers to take a personal interest in any one individual. Most schools do have tutor schemes, or counselling, or some form of support for each young person, but parents should never assume that this will meet all their teenager's needs. Adolescents need to know that there is someone who has a special concern for their welfare. That is the responsibility of parents.

Society

The second half of the twentieth century has seen a revolution in sexual attitudes and sexual behaviour. While this is not the place to enter into an extended analysis of the reasons for these changes,

TEENAGERS AND SEXUALITY

it is important to note some of the effects, especially as they concern young people.

The first thing to look at is the contraceptive pill. The pill has, since the late 1960s, been available to any woman who wants it. This fact has resulted in the separation of sexual behaviour from procreation, for the first time in history. The impact of this cannot be overestimated. Initially the effect was felt by married women, who became able to control the timing of their pregnancies, and plan childbirth in a way that had never been possible before. In due course, however, more widespread effects became apparent. Men and women experienced greater sexual freedom, both within marriage, and outside it. Not surprisingly the possibilities of sexual experimentation and sexual licence were not lost on the young. It was this new found freedom which, in part, led to the now famous – or infamous – permissiveness of the 1960s.

Another major change has had to do with the public acceptability of sexual material. Today no film is complete without an erotic, usually explicit, love scene. Much advertising depends on the use of sexual imagery. TV soaps compete to include sexual violence, underage sex, and so on. Teenage magazines appear to cover nothing but sexual matters. The f-word, once unacceptable in the paperback version of 'Lady Chatterley's Lover', is now so common as to be hardly noticeable.

It is said that we live in an 'eroticised' society, where sex is everywhere. It is even said that there are no taboos left where sex is concerned, whereas we shall see this is not in fact the case. What is certainly true, however, is that the social changes that have occurred since the 1960s have had far-reaching effects on young people's lives.

The most obvious consequence for teenagers is that they cannot get away from sex. It is pervasive. Adults, who are more mature, may have better defences. They may be able to filter out what they don't want to hear. They may also have better control over their responses to sexual messages. For teenagers, who have less maturity, less sexual experience, and higher levels of anxiety

LEARNING ABOUT SEX

about sexual matters anyway, this is not so easy. Although this is something that is rarely discussed, it should be a matter of concern. The fact that there is so much sex on public display is bound to create greater sexual arousal. Are we providing young people with the skills and resources to cope with this? I suspect not.

As a result of all this it is not surprising to find that teenagers feel themselves under pressure to become sexually active. It is all too easy to gain the impression that 'everyone is doing it'. From this it is but a simple step to the conclusion that, if everyone else is doing it, and you are not, then there must be something wrong with you. Pressures upon young people stem from friends and from the wider peer group. These pressures may be quite open and direct. However, there is also a range of subtle and indirect pressures, including those created by the media and by the values of our culture. One of these values has to do with the right to expect sexual gratification. How could young people not be influenced by such an expectation?

> A friend of mine did it with a boy when she was 13.
> She said "Oh you must, you must". I listened
> because I was very influenced by other people, and
> she was my best friend and I had to do what she said
> or I wasn't in with her. I used to make it up that I
> did, but I didn't. So I didn't until I was 16, which
> was still quite young, but just so I could be in with
> my friends.
>
> (18-year-old girl)

There has been an unhealthy tendency among some groups of adults in Western societies to blame the young for what is called 'sexual permissiveness'. Such a tendency is both shortsighted and hypocritical. The young – by this we mean adolescents – do not set trends, they follow them. Young people are influenced in their behaviour primarily by what they see around them. Where sexuality is concerned, they learn from parents and neighbours. They learn from aunts, uncles, teachers and politicians – in short, they learn from adults.

I call this 'invisible learning', because it does not involve lessons and textbooks. Neither does it involve any direct instruction or guidance. Invisible learning is what is absorbed by people through watching and listening to what is going on around them. Since sex is an important subject, young people are especially sensitive to the way adults behave in this domain. Furthermore sex is a mystery, a puzzle that needs to be solved. Children have numerous unanswered questions. Many of these questions will, in the end, be answered by observing adults. It is worth remembering that young people learn from adults, not the other way around.

Friends

It is common knowledge that young people learn as much about sex, if not more, from their friends than from anyone else. On the whole, adults tend to be suspicious of this learning. It is assumed that what teenagers learn from their friends consists mainly of false or misleading information. It is also assumed that it is through friends and the peer group that myths about sexuality circulate (such as 'you can't get pregnant if you do it standing up').

Very little research evidence is available on this topic, so in fact we don't really know much about what might be called 'playground learning'. It seems probable that there are both good and bad aspects of this. We certainly need to recognise that friends have a very important part to play in helping young people to piece together the puzzle of sex.

Let us look first at the positive aspects of playground learning.

- Young people are less inhibited with friends. This makes it possible for them to share anxieties and concerns, and to discuss difficult topics.

LEARNING ABOUT SEX

- Young people obtain support from each other. It is easier to talk about an embarrassing or awkward topic with someone if you know they are facing the same problems.
- The peer group is a social arena. This means that some learning will take place through trying out different ways of behaving. Much learning about sex will take place, not by talking or listening, but by interacting with others, and discovering what works and what doesn't.

Of course learning from friends is not always a good thing. It is certainly true that young people do not have all the facts. They may lack information, or they may simply get things wrong. It is easy to see how one person's misunderstanding can get passed around a group of friends, thus magnifying the effect of ignorance.

> *When I was in my primary school – I was about ten – we started sex education for the first time, which I thought was good really starting in primary school. And you know, friends were talking about things on telly and that and they were going around talking about periods and that in the playground. They were saying one can last for about six months and all this lot. And you were getting really confused and going home and telling your mum all about this. I always remember being told that you got pregnant by a seed being put in a cup. That's how you got pregnant. So I got a bit confused over that, because I thought that for about two or three years. I wouldn't tell anyone that. I really felt embarrassed about that sort of thing. But that happens a lot. I know from my friends as well as they have told me that that happens.*
> *(16-year-old girl)*

Perhaps the most damaging feature of playground learning is social pressure. I have already given an example of young people believing that they ought to be sexually active, because it appears that so many of their friends are gaining sexual experience. Young people boast about and exaggerate the extent of their sexual activity, but the effect is to create pressure on many teenagers to hurry up and get on with it.

We need to understand more about the role of friends in the area of sexual learning. Friends can be an asset, a strength and a resource for young people. As adults we need to identify more clearly the ways in which incorrect information gets passed around. This would then make it easier for teachers and parents to counteract the effects, and to provide essential knowledge at key stages of development. Lastly, adults could help young people to resist social pressure by providing support, as well as by supplying the factual information the teenagers need to help them stand up to the peer group.

The media

Few subjects have caused more disagreement than the effects of the media on children and young people. Once again this is a debate where, unfortunately, only the extreme positions receive much attention. Furthermore most of the argument has revolved around the effects of violence, and little note has been taken of the effect of the media on the sexual attitudes and behaviour of the young.

It is clear that children and adolescents are receptive to, and are therefore likely to learn from, all aspects of the media. Here we must include not only TV and newspapers, but also magazines films, videos and books. The big question is – what sort of learning takes place? Do young people absorb everything they watch and read? Are they prepared to believe whatever appears on television This is what adults fear. However, there may be an alternative view. Perhaps young people are actually quite discriminating Maybe they are only too well aware that television is television not real life. It is possible that they are quite skilled at sorting ou

LEARNING ABOUT SEX

what is rubbish from what is useful. If this is the case, then perhaps the influence of the media is not so bad after all.

In fact the truth probably lies somewhere in between these two positions. Age and maturity have something to do with it, for obviously the older the individual the more discriminating they are. In addition it is probably true to say that people are more influenced by the media if they do not have alternative sources of information. Thus, for example, young people who have good sex education at school, as well as the chance to discuss sexual issues at home with their parents, will be better able to judge the accuracy of media information. Lastly books, videos and magazines do not all carry the same weight. Information from a respected agony aunt in *Just Seventeen* is more likely to be believed than something one girl tells another in *Coronation Street*.

As with all sources of learning, there are advantages and disadvantages to the media. Some of the benefits are:

- Difficult topics can be addressed by responsible journalists and TV producers. In Britain there have been examples of soaps such as *Brookside* dealing with topics which are not dealt with anywhere else.
- Agony aunts and uncles do provide information on topics which teachers and parents find difficult to tackle. Judging by the stream of letters and queries reaching these journalists, they are offering an important service to many thousands of young people.
- As with all things, learning gained from the media has to be placed in context. If media information is all that is available, this cannot be good. However, if it is one element of a wider picture, then the encouragement of imagination, the opportunity to learn about different worlds and different values, and the ability to compare one's own experiences with those of other people all enhance the young person's learning.

In conclusion we need to acknowledge that the media can have a powerful influence on young people. However, the extent of that influence depends on a number of factors. It is up to parents and other adults to ensure:

- that different media are on offer. Sitting in front of the television day in and day out is not good for anyone. Books, films and magazines all provide alternative viewpoints
- that the young person develops the ability to make judgements about what he or she is watching or reading. This skill can be developed by adults at home and at school
- that the young person is not continually alone when exposed to the media. Any influence the media may have is undoubtedly diminished if the young person has the opportunity to discuss the material with others. Parents and other trusted adults are obviously of greatest importance in this respect.

Communication

This chapter is concerned with the way young people learn about sex. As we have seen, learning takes place in all sorts of ways, and stems from many different sources. In spite of this, it still remains true that the most powerful learning occurs as a result of communication between people. In the case of teenagers and sex, one critical aspect of communication is that which involves parents.

Research shows that, almost without exception, young people want more chances to talk with adults about sex and sexuality. When asked with which adults they would most like to discuss these matters, the great majority say their parents. If this is the case, why don't they? Because, as young people see it, their parents are too embarrassed or awkward to make such discussions possible.

Strangely, adults have a rather different perspective! The experience of most parents is that it is the teenagers who are the more embarrassed by the topic of sex. It is the youngsters who hold back, or find some excuse, or end up by saying 'don't bother, mum, I know it all already'. So, what can be done? First, a few things about communication.

Not all communication is verbal communication

You don't necessarily have to talk to someone to communicate with them. You can communicate your interest and concern to your children in many different ways. Leaving a good sex education book or information leaflet lying around the house is one way of saying 'I want to help'. A squeeze on the shoulder when someone is upset, or simply an offer to go to the clinic or doctor together – these are types of communication which may be more effective than saying 'okay –time to talk!'.

Verbal communication is complicated, and involves a lot more than talking

Good communication is often described as a 'two-way street'. By this it is meant that if you want to communicate with someone, you have to listen as well as talk. Your teenager will be far more likely to concentrate on what you have to say if he or she knows that you are also prepared to listen. Listening and talking go hand in hand. Closely linked with this is a third communication skill – making sure you have been heard. After all, there's not much point in spending ten minutes reeling off a whole list of arguments to support your point of view, if the other person cannot hear what you have to say. In order to be heard you have to choose the right time to express your opinion, you have to use an appropriate tone and language, and, most important of all, you have to show that you are willing to listen to the other person too.

Understanding the skills of communication will help in overcoming some of the embarrassment of talking about sex. If you want to be able to communicate with your teenager about sex, or indeed about any difficult topic, here are some dos and don'ts.

TEENAGERS AND SEXUALITY

Don't   expect to sit down at the kitchen table and say 'Right, let's talk about the facts of life'. It won't work.

Do   be prepared to wait for the right time. This may be after a family event, a scene from TV, or when your daughter has had a row with her boyfriend.

Don't   try to cover all the issues at the same time. Take it slowly. Remember, there *will* be other opportunities, as long as you don't force the pace.

Do   be prepared to share some of your own experiences. It is helpful for young people to learn that their parents didn't get it right the first time either.

Don't   go too far with this sort of disclosure. Your son or daughter wants to know you're human, not that you've had a superhuman sex life!

Do   be prepared to make yourself available, even at inconvenient times. Teenagers are more likely to want to talk at midnight than at midday. This can be hard for parents, especially for those who have a long day ahead. Nonetheless some 'heart to heart' talks are too important to be missed.

Don't   try to set the agenda yourself. Listen carefully to the clues that your teenager provides. He or she will find a way of telling you what's important at any particular time. You are more likely to be able to communicate about the subjects on the teenager's agenda, than about those on your own agenda.

Do   be prepared to help with setting the boundaries of acceptable behaviour. Teenagers may need you to help them sort out how far to go in their sexual behaviour. Be honest, and tell them what you think the limits are. This may come as a great relief to them.

Finally,

Do   show your teenager some respect. Good communication is based on the belief that the other person is genuinely interested in who you are, and what you have to say. If you can get that across to your son or daughter there will be opportunities for genuine sharing between you.

Useful reading

Let's Talk About Sex by Robie Harris, Walker Books 1994. This book provides open and comprehensive answers to the questions young people ask about conception, puberty, birth control, AIDS, the body, families and sexual health.

You and Your Adolescent by Larry Steinberg and Anne Levine, Vermillion 1992.

Useful organisations

For information about sex education in schools, contact **The Sex Education Forum**, 8 Wakley Street, London EC1V 7QE. Tel: 0171 843 6051/6052.

CHAPTER THREE

Sexual development in early adolescence

In this chapter I wish to consider some aspects of sexual development which start to occur either during or after puberty. The topics I want to cover here include:

- the need for privacy
- relationships with adults
- boys and girls are different
- masturbation
- the fears and anxieties of adults
- the fears and anxieties of teenagers.

The need for privacy

One almost universal feature of teenage behaviour, especially during or following puberty, is the need for greater privacy. It is at this time that parents notice doors being locked, signs appearing which

SEXUAL DEVELOPMENT IN EARLY ADOLESCENCE

say 'no admittance', and longer queues for the bathroom. For some parents this can seem like an unwelcome change. Suddenly your son or daughter , once an open, loving child with whom you could discuss anything at all, becomes a closed private individual. You feel shut out, and this is an experience which can be very hurtful.

It is important to keep in mind that there are good reasons behind the need for privacy.

- **Sensitivity about bodily changes**   Young people may find the physical changes of puberty very unsettling. They may feel shy or awkward or embarrassed. As a result they want to be sure that no one barges into the bedroom or bathroom while they are undressed.
- **Self-consciousness**   At this stage teenagers become hypersensitive about their appearance. They may want to try out different hairstyles, or different clothes, and they may want to do this on their own. The mirror can become their best friend.
- **Sexuality**   The need for privacy may be related to the existence of new sexual feelings or fantasies. Your teenager may stick pictures of pop stars on his or her bedroom walls, or read teenage magazines secretly in bed. Young people need space and time alone to experience these early signs of sexuality.

While parents may find this need for privacy difficult to cope with, it is important to remember that it is an essential part of growing up,. Teenagers do need space and time on their own. They do need to be allowed to have some privacy. Without it they will feel pressured and harassed.

It may seem to parents that the need for privacy is a sign that the child is lost to them, or doing something that has been forbidden. In fact quite the opposite is true. Young people who are allowed some private space will be more likely to seek out their parents when they need them. Teenagers who feel that their parents are always intruding are the ones who move away as soon as it is possible to do so.

> She often says to me "Why don't you talk about your problems?" I say "I do, I just don't talk to you. I talk to my friends". I have talked to my mum about things but not at the time they're happening. I tell her about them after they've happened, after I sorted it out for myself what's happening. I still think she wants me to tell her, but I can't.
>
> *(15-year-old girl)*

Relationships with adults

Adults, and especially parents, have a major role to play in the life of the teenager. A supportive and concerned parent can make all the difference when a young person is unhappy or upset. A sensitive teacher can provide a lifeline when things seem very bleak. An aunt, uncle or other relative can offer advice or information which enables the young person to solve a pressing personal problem. These are just a few examples of ways in which adults can be influential at key moments.

More generally, though, adults matter to adolescents for a number of reasons:

- However much bravado there is, young people are still dependent on adults for many of their emotional needs.
- Teenagers need boundaries and structure. They need to know how far they can go. Only adults can provide these boundaries.
- Young people need role models. As they face questions about their identity teenagers need models and examples upon which to base their choices.
- Adolescents need a reference point. Research shows that, as

far as self-image is concerned, young people are more
influenced by how their parents judge them than by any
other factor.
- Teenagers need encouragement and support. Apart from
  intelligence, the factor which has most influence on
  academic performance is parental interest and involvement
  in schoolwork.

Some parents may find the proposition 'adults do matter' difficult to believe. Faced with a moody, resentful, withdrawn 14-year-
old, it may seem that the very opposite is true. Nonetheless you
are important. You do make a difference. Your teenager needs you
just as much as he or she did in early childhood. It is only that the
needs are expressed in different ways – often heavily disguised!

Not surprisingly adults find moodiness and irritability difficult to
deal with. Sometimes parents say that their child's behaviour simply doesn't make sense. Teenagers seem to be a sort of Jekyll and
Hyde – sunny and smiling one moment, impossible the next. It is
worth remembering that behaviour of this sort is very common
among young people, especially in the early years of adolescence.
Here are some of the reasons:

- **Hormones**   During puberty a major change takes place in
  your adolescent's hormonal balance. Adjusting to these
  alterations is not easy, as we have already noted. Some
  moodiness is probably a direct result of hormonal variation.
- **Transition**   Your adolescent faces a difficult task – moving
  from childhood to adulthood over a long drawn-out period.
  During much of this time they won't know quite where they
  stand. Mature or immature? Grown up or child-like? Much
  of the puzzling behaviour reflects this uncertainty.
- **Breaking away**   Another challenge faced by your
  adolescent is that they need to create more of an emotional
  distance from you. This is a natural part of growing up.
  Nonetheless breaking away is never easy, and sometimes
  teenagers may seem to overreact. They may give the

impression of wanting to reject you altogether. Keep in mind that this is only a stage. It is no more than a strategy to help them with the task of moving away.

We need to understand a little bit about adolescent development, and the important role that adults play at this stage if we are to make sense of adolescent sexuality. Sexuality is an especially sensitive topic. It is a central feature of development at this time. Yet it is a subject fraught with embarrassment and anxiety. Young people need information, advice, support and the opportunity to discuss many of the issues associated with sexuality, and yet it may seem to be impossible for them to explore this topic with their parents.

Many of the points outlined in the previous sections are relevant here. Adults are very important indeed where sexuality is concerned and yet teenage behaviour may seem to suggest the opposite. It is up to parents to overcome the barriers, and recognise the role they can play. It is possible to provide information and advice, it is possible to be supportive, and it is possible to have an influence. Parents can be active and involved, and we will be looking at how this can be done in subsequent chapters of this book.

Boys and girls are different

This may seem to be stating the obvious, but it is necessary to underline the fact that early sexual development is experienced quite differently by males and females. Many parents reading this will have both sons and daughters. Yet, surprisingly, and all too frequently, families fail to appreciate that the needs of boys and girls are not going to be the same. The difference in gender has important implications, requiring different approaches, and sensitivity on the part of parents to the characteristics of masculine and feminine development. Let me outline some of these characteristics:

- The physical changes associated with puberty may have more of an impact on girls than on boys. Certainly boys do not have to adjust to any experience equivalent to menstruation.
- Girls express greater dissatisfaction with their bodies than boys do during early adolescence. Feelings of dissatisfaction for girls centre particularly on breast size, weight, and facial characteristics.
- Girls feel that they are the target of more media pressure than boys, in relation to what constitutes ideal weight, height and shape. There is more stereotyping of female beauty, and girls are under more pressure than boys to diet and to conform to what is considered to be 'the perfect woman'.
- Girls' and boys' friendships are different. Boys' friendships are centred on shared activities, while girls are more likely to have close relationships in which feelings can be discussed.
- Girls get more support from their friends in this way. This is especially important, since boys have less opportunity to express emotion. They may therefore be more vulnerable when things go wrong.
- Boys are more likely to be affected by the lack of appropriate role models. The fact that so much parenting is done by mothers does put boys at a disadvantage. Where there is an absence of a close relationship with an adult male the boy's developing sexuality may suffer.
- Parents are more likely to be worried about the personal safety of girls than of boys. This can result in girls experiencing greater restrictions on their freedom, which is a cause of considerable conflict in some families.
- Finally, the distribution of power in sexual relationships is

still unequal. This means that in many situations it remains difficult for girls to take control of events. This has particular relevance to the use of contraceptives, and to decisions and choices about how far to go in sexual activity.

These issues will not necessarily apply in all circumstances. Nonetheless if parents can keep in mind the differing needs of boys and girls, they will undoubtedly be more likely to be meeting the needs of all the teenagers in their family.

> ❝ I think up until puberty for girls there's this wonderful feeling that you can climb anywhere, run anywhere, do anything you like and then you're brought up short by this equipment that starts changing and slows you down and makes you weepy and bleeds on you and it goes out of your control ... A lot of girls around eleven, they actually can run faster than boys and they're more verbal and they're cheeky and they feel they can do anything and suddenly you know, shutters come down about what's possible on certain days of the month. I think that's something that has to be talked about to girls in order for them to place it and allow it to happen to them without allowing it to stop them doing things they still want to do. ❞
>
> (Mother of two daughters)

Masturbation

Masturbation is a topic that is rarely discussed. It is unlikely to feature in any sex education lesson, and it is hardly ever mentioned by parents when talking to their children. Indeed it is even one of the few subjects that is avoided when young people are with their friends. Why should this be so?

SEXUAL DEVELOPMENT IN EARLY ADOLESCENCE

It has to be concluded that strong taboos still operate where masturbation is concerned. How many couples, I wonder, have discussed the subject with each other? It is not quite clear why masturbation is such a difficult topic. Is it simply a hangover from the Victorian era? Is it because attaining sexual gratification on your own is still in some way seen as shameful? Masturbation is certainly a good example of the fact that, although there have been huge changes in sexual attitudes and behaviour since the 1960s, there are still some areas in which substantial inhibitions remain.

Masturbation is a perfectly normal and healthy expression of sexual need. It is a pleasurable activity which has no harmful or negative consequences. Surveys of sexual behaviour show that there is wide variation between individuals in the frequency of masturbation. Some masturbate often, some rarely, some not at all. Approximately two-thirds of women have masturbated some time or another while almost all men have done so. Many people masturbate at the same time as having a satisfying sex life with a partner.

There are still many myths about masturbation, and teenagers are more likely than adults to worry about some of these. No one any longer believes Victorian notions such as that masturbation leads to blindness. Nonetheless many people still do have anxieties about it. Boys may fear that masturbation will affect their virility or their capacity to produce semen. Girls may worry that their clitoris or vagina will become less responsive to stimulation when they have sex with another person. Both boys and girls may feel ashamed that they have become aroused on their own, rather than with a partner.

Young people need reassurance about masturbation. They need to know that it is healthy and harmless. They also need to know that it is something that most people do at some stage in their lives. Masturbation is a normal outlet for sexual arousal. If adults have the opportunity they should make sure that teenagers know the facts about this subject.

The fears and anxieties of parents

I want to conclude this chapter by outlining some of the most common fears experienced by both adults and teenagers in relation to adolescent sexuality. All of us have worries and anxieties and one useful way to deal with these is to be open and honest about them. Let us first look at the parents' perspective.

Talking about sex encourages teenagers to go and try it

Many adults worry that sex education, or discussions in the home, act as a green light for young people to go out and experiment. This is an understandable concern, but the facts indicate that the opposite is true. The most conclusive evidence comes from comparisons of teenage pregnancy rates in different countries. Where teenage pregnancy rates are lowest there is extensive sex education, and freely available contraceptive services for young people – as in Holland and Sweden. Furthermore, research in Britain and the United States indicates that young people are more likely to delay their first sexual experience if they come from a home where sex is discussed openly. If you still have doubts remember this. Sex is a topic of public debate. Your teenager is going to be talking about it anyway. Isn't it better he or she talks about it with you?

Sex is too embarrassing to discuss

Many people are too embarrassed to discuss sex, especially with their own children. However there are many ways of communicating, and not all of them involve sitting down and talking. Suggestions for different approaches to communication have already been outlined in the previous chapter.

Your teenager may know more than you

This is a possibility, particularly in relation to topics such as HIV/AIDS or drugs. Since the mid 1980s school sex education has concentrated on the topic of AIDS, which has meant that many young people are better informed than their parents. Be honest, and be prepared to accept that you are not the fountain of all wisdom! If you make it clear to your son or daughter that you are keen to learn, they will be only too happy to share their knowledge with you. They will also then be more likely to take on board what you have to teach them.

Your son or daughter will get involved in a sexual relationship before he or she is ready

There is little a parent can do to stop a young person becoming sexually active if that is what they are determined to do. However there is an enormous amount a parent can do to make sure that the teenager is well informed, and properly prepared. This applies both to physical and emotional preparation for sex. Parents can also ensure that boys and girls have access to an appropriate contraceptive. In summary, you can't stop them doing it, but you can help them to be safe.

Your son or daughter will be subjected to peer pressure from unsuitable friends

Peer pressure is a powerful force which operates among young people. However, some teenagers are more able to resist pressure than others, and it is quite clear that adults play a clear role here. Research shows that support from parents is the one thing which is most helpful to young people in resisting peer pressure. Try not to criticise your children's friends, or exclude them from your home. The more they are part of your life, the more influence you will have, and the more likely you are to be able to keep an eye on what's going on.

The fears and anxieties of teenagers

Finally, let us look at some of the fears of young people themselves. If you as a parent can be aware of these, there may be situations in which you can help.

'My body is not normal'

This is probably the most common fear of all. In fact there are few teenagers who have not worried at some time or other about their bodies, and how they compare with their friends. Two things are worth bearing in mind here:

- First, everyone is different. There is no such thing as normal where bodies are concerned. People develop at different rates, and in different ways. No two girls have exactly the same breasts. No two boys have exactly the same penises. Your son or daughter does not need to worry about being different.
- Second, the way we develop around puberty bears very little relation to how we are as mature adults. Whether your teenager is slow or fast in his or her development will be forgotten within a few years. It may feel very important to your teenager to be in step with the rest of the class. This is understandable. In the long-term, however, the differences between friends at 12 or 13 will have completely disappeared by the age of 16 or 18.

'I think about sex too much'

Many young people find that, as they move into adolescence, the subject of sex begins to dominate their thinking. As with everything to do with sex, there are great differences between individuals. Some young people may spend a lot of their time having daydreams or fantasies about sexual matters. They may lie in bed thinking sexual thoughts, they may masturbate, or they may seek out books or videos having sexual themes. On the other hand there are others of the same age who do none of these things.

There is no such thing as thinking about sex too much. We all have different levels of sexual need, and different levels of arousal. Each of us has to come to terms with the way we are, and find healthy and satisfactory outlets for our sexual desires.

'Should I have done "it" by now?'

In our society there is considerable pressure on young people to become sexually active. This pressure comes from the media, from the adult world, and it also comes from the peer group. There is also undoubtedly much exaggeration, by both boys and girls, about the extent of their sexual experience. Nonetheless many feel that they need to have done certain things in order to 'keep in with the crowd'. This can create powerful pressures, and make life very uncomfortable for some young people.

Two things can help teenagers to resist peer pressure:

* Having access to good sensible information about sexuality. For example it helps young people to know that less than one in five 16-year-old girls has had sexual intercourse in Britain today. In some parts of the country this figure is as low as one in eight.
* As I have already indicated, support from parents is crucial in enabling the young person to resist peer pressure. If adolescents know that their parents respect and value them, and if they know that help will be available if it is needed then they are likely to have the strength and confidence to stand up for what they believe in.

'Am I too easily aroused'/'Am I frigid?'

It is not surprising that adolescents worry about their ability to become sexually aroused. After all, sexual experiences will be quite new to them, and young people are bound to be uncertain about how their bodies function, and whether what is happening to them is the same as what is happening to everyone else.

Many boys find getting an erection extremely embarrassing, especially if it occurs in public. Boys may be surprised at how easily they become excited, and alarmed that this can occur on a bus, in a school lesson, or on the street corner. Sexual arousal for girls is much less visible, and so there may be different fears. Even so, early experiences of erect nipples or of becoming wet around the vaginal area may be worrying too. Girls may feel convinced that such things are visible, even if they are not.

Anxieties about frigidity or impotence are also commonplace, being directly linked to questions of sexual performance. Boys may worry that they won't be able to do 'it', and will thus become a laughing stock; girls may worry that unless they are sexually responsive they will be unable to attract or hold on to a boyfriend. In most cases fears of this sort recede as young people become sexually experienced. Where they persist some help or advice may be necessary. Suitable organisations are listed at the end of this chapter.

> ❛ I remember I was quite worried before. You know, when you sort of lose your virginity you think "I've got to put on a big, a good show". And then when you actually do get round to it, you usually blow it very quickly and you think "Is this it? Is this what it's all about?". Worrying that the girl has probably done it before, and thinks you're an absolute failure, and she's gonna tell everyone, and that all goes through your head. It's all that macho kind of thing, that you've got to be able to perform, you've got to be you know big and hard and tough and all this kind of rubbish. ❜
>
> (19-year-old boy)

'Am I gay, lesbian or straight?'

It is a tragedy that in our society we are unable to talk openly about issues to do with sexual orientation. We ought to be able to offer young people information and advice about heterosexuality and homosexuality, as well as the opportunity to discuss any concerns they may have. Sadly we cannot do so, and thus questions about sexual orientation go unanswered. Although we cannot be sure, it is probable that many heterosexual young people worry at some stage if they are gay or lesbian. Similarly those who are homosexual worry about their future, how their parents and friends will react, and so on. We do urgently need a more responsible and sensitive approach to this topic. I say more about this topic in Chapter 7.

Useful reading

Adolescence: The Survival Guide for Parents by E Fenwick and T Smith, Kindersley 1993. A good book which looks at how to improve communications between parents and teenagers. It includes case studies of families with young people.

Teenagers and Sexuality This pack is produced by the Trust for the Study of Adolescence. It considers a variety of issues to do with adolescent sexuality, and includes an audiotape of parents and teenagers talking about the issues. Available from TSA Publishing Ltd, 23 New Road, Brighton, East Sussex BN1 1WZ. Tel: 01273 693311.

CHAPTER FOUR

First relationships

In this chapter I want to begin to explore the issues associated with early sexual relationships. Clearly the first time an individual experiences sex represents a major landmark. It is something we all remember vividly, and for most it symbolises an important step towards adulthood. The idea of 'losing one's virginity' can represent a scary event, an obstacle to be overcome, a challenge, a longed-for moment. Boys and girls may well feel differently about it, but one thing is certain – for most in our society it is the closest we come to having a rite of passage – a ritual that marks the fact that we have, at last, reached maturity. Early sexuality is also likely to involve a whole range of new feelings and experiences. Understanding and support from parents at this time can be crucial. In this chapter I want to cover:

- love and romance
- readiness for sex
- contraception
- personal safety
- essential messages for parents to emphasise.

FIRST RELATIONSHIPS

Love and romance

There are many many different ways in which a first sexual relationship can happen. In most cases – even today – young people do not start to have sex until they are in love, or until they feel something special for their partner. While the general impression given by the media is that teenagers of all ages are spending most of their time hopping in and out of bed with anyone they fancy, the facts are rather different. The great majority of teenagers:

- have sex within a lasting relationship
- have sex with only one person at a time
- believe sex should only be part of an important relationship.

Most recent figures in Britain show that by the age of 16 only 20 per cent of girls (one in five) have had sexual intercourse, while approximately 25 per cent of boys of this age are sexually experienced. These figures are higher than they were 10 or 20 years ago, and there has therefore been a gradual lowering of the age of first sexual activity. It is clear, therefore, that young people are having sex at an earlier age than they were in the 1960s or the 1970s.

In spite of this, however, the figures are still lower than many people imagine. Put another way, the figures show that by the age of 16 four out of five girls (or 80 per cent) have not had a first sexual experience. Thus the overwhelming majority of girls at 16 are still virgins in Britain today. This is not the sort of headline usually seen in the tabloid newspapers! It should also be noted that there are marked regional variations. While in some inner city areas the figures may be higher than this, in other parts of the country fewer than one in eight 16-year-old girls have started being sexually active. These facts are important, and help us to get some perspective on an issue about which many people become very emotional.

Research shows that for most young people – although not all – their first sexual experience happens only after a lengthy sequence of other events. First, two young people start to see each other regularly. They may go out together, or spend time together at the weekend. They begin to share hopes and ideas with each other and, if things progress, they begin to develop a feeling that this is a special relationship. At the same time that all this is happening they may begin to be affectionate with each other. They may hold hands, or kiss, and want to be physically close to each other. This may lead to further sexual exploration, which may be accompanied by the first sense of 'being in love'.

> I've got a friend who's 13 at the moment who's quite a good friend. She always tends to act much older, but she's 13 and she always sort of goes out with a boy and sort of a week later she'll go "I'm in love" and she'll be serious and I sort of laugh at her really. I know that a week later she'll have given up on him and go out with another boy. Lots of times in adolescence feelings can come out a lot more and it can make you feel like there's something there, like love or something, even after only a week of going out with somebody. So it takes quite a long time to settle down and sort of realise that not every little feeling is love. It might just be lust or you know friendship or something like that in a different way. It takes quite a while to get that sorted out.
> *(15-year-old girl)*

Of course young people may believe they are in love with someone without any physical contact having occurred. Alternatively sexual activity may take place without there being any special feelings between two people. For some the first sexual experience may happen at a party, when both have had too much to drink.

However, in most cases early sexual behaviour does take place in the context of a developing relationship, and it is especially important for parents to be aware of this. In a moment we shall consider how parents should respond, and what role they have to play. If parents see teenagers as being sexually promiscuous, wanting simply to have as much sex as possible, then their judgements will be affected by this viewpoint. I can only recommend that you listen carefully to your own teenager. You will be most likely to find that he or she believes sex to be something which should only be part of a meaningful relationship.

In any event, if you are not sure what your son or daughter's views are, why not ask? You may have an unexpectedly interesting discussion.

Readiness for sex

Young people today grow up in a world where attitudes to sex are very confusing indeed. As I have indicated in Chapter 2, from their early years children are trying to make sense of the puzzle of sex: 'What is it all about?'

A hundred years ago – or even 50 years ago – sex was much less of an issue. It was for making babies, and for the most part took place within marriage. Nowadays these answers no longer make sense. So what is the meaning of sex? Is it no more than a pleasurable activity, rather like having a good meal? Does it matter if it has nothing to do with love, or trust, or commitment to another person? Can sex be as good with a stranger as with a long-term partner? These are the sorts of questions young people are bound to ask. Unfortunately the answers are far from clear.

As I have indicated, it is to adults that young people look for solutions to the puzzle. What do they see? They see many families disrupted by divorce or separation, often because one partner falls in love with someone else. They see neighbours, relatives, public figures having affairs. They see adults openly disagreeing about things like sex education, the provision of contraceptives for young people, and so on.

The effect of all this must be:

- to create uncertainty
- to underline the fact that many adults will sacrifice an enormous amount for sexual gratification
- to lead young people to question whether adults have any authority to give them advice
- to conclude that they need to make their own decisions about the meaning of sex.

I raise these issues because one of the questions most frequently asked by young people is 'When is someone ready to have sex?' It is one of the most difficult to answer, but also, it is one that cannot be answered without having some view on the meaning of sex.

After all, if you think sex is simply about bodily pleasure, then young people might as well have sex for fun, whenever they feel like it. Of course, very few of us take such a view. Most of us believe that sex should be delayed at least until the individual is emotionally mature enough to take precautions and cope with the consequences. Indeed most parents would probably say that they hope their son or daughter would wait for as long as possible. Some may believe that sex should only take place once two people are engaged, or at least intending to get married. Today this is a minority view, but it is certainly not uncommon.

> Well, I'm Christian so technically I should say you should not have sex until after marriage, but I also don't believe in hard and fast social rules, so I think the most sensible thing to say is when you feel ready and comfortable. For me I think that would be when I'd left home. While I'm still at home I still feel too much, even though sort of technically old enough and all the rest of it I still feel too much part of a family and a child within that family. So I think it's important to get it right. I mean, when you feel ready, and when you think y··· are old enough.
>
> *(16-year-old girl)*

FIRST RELATIONSHIPS

For complicated reasons the sexual activity of our children is something most adults find difficult to deal with. It helps to be aware of some of our complex feelings, especially our reluctance to accept the sexuality of our sons and daughters. As adults we need to acknowledge our own strong feelings if the advice we give to young people is to be of any use at all.

So, what do you say when you are asked 'Mum, how old do I have to be before I can have sex?'. To some extent the answer to this depends on the values of the parents. Some may say 'Not until you've left home' or 'Not until you're engaged'. The danger here, of course, is that any message which sounds like 'I don't want you to do it' may act as a challenge or provocation. When they ask this question young people do not want to be told that sex is forbidden to them. If this is what they hear it may be just the signal they need to go off and try it.

What teenagers do want is an open and honest discussion about early sexual activity. This should be combined with a recognition that at 16, 15 or even 14, they are old enough to have sex, and there is not much that can stop them if they are really determined.

This may sound depressing to parents who worry about their teenagers' health, safety and welfare. However, there are many ways in which parents can be helpful. There is much that parents can do to emphasise the risks of early sexual activity, and there are strong reasons why young people should delay. Outlining these in a non-judgemental fashion can make a real difference.

These are some the things that you can say:

- You should not have sex until you feel sure you can trust the other person.
- You should not have sex until *you* feel ready. If the other person is putting pressure on you – then say no.
- You should not have sex until you can discuss and decide about contraception together.
- You should not have sex until you can handle the emotional feelings that you may experience.

- You should not have sex until you are absolutely sure you and your partner will be protected against pregnancy and STDs (sexually transmitted diseases).

These answers do not cover every eventuality. They will certainly not provide a foolproof guide for a young person concerned about this issue. They will however be helpful, and will certainly lead to further questioning about the meaning of 'trust', 'emotional maturity' and so on. At the very least they will show that sex and relationships are linked up together. If expressed in the right way these points will encourage your son or daughter to stop and think.

Contraception

It is sometimes very difficult for parents to be clear as to their role in relation to contraception. How far can parents go in trying to make sure that a teenager is going to use the right contraceptive? Should a father buy condoms for his son? Should a mother take her daughter to the GP, or the family planning clinic?

> I remember when I wanted to go on the pill, it took me weeks and weeks to ask my mum. I remember I was like waiting for the right moment for weeks like, and she eventually just said "yeah, all right then, I'll take you down the family planning clinic". And I was going aaaagh! I had to wait till we went on holiday and wait till my mum was a bit drunk and after we'd had a meal to eventually ask her but she was fine about it. It's embarrassing.
>
> *(18-year-old girl)*

The fact is that parents are caught in a trap here. If they try and help with contraception they may believe they are encouraging sexual activity, or they may fear being accused of interfering in something that is private. On the other hand, if they don't do anything, they experience all the anxiety of not being sure that the teenager is taking the proper precautions.

It is my view that parents do have a role, and a very important one. Reasons that parents give themselves for not doing anything are often excuses, as we can see if we look at them more closely.

To give advice about contraception will encourage sexual behaviour

There is absolutely no evidence that this is the case. To think like this is to assume that there are no other influences on young people. Your teenager will be worrying about these questions, and looking around for advice, whether you give it or not. Isn't it better that the advice comes from you, rather than from someone else?

To give advice about contraception is to intrude upon something that is private

Whether this is the case or not depends entirely upon how the subject is approached. If the parent tries to take over, treating the teenager as an irresponsible child, it will not go down too well! If the parent treads cautiously, offering advice and support when and if the young person wants it, then this is likely to be more acceptable.

The question of contraception is a difficult one for young people. They do need assistance to get it right. While some find their way to user-friendly clinics where they can have a full and frank discussion with a family planning nurse, these young people are probably in the minority. More often teenagers do not find it easy to get good advice, and it is here that parents can play such a key role. Questions young people are likely to have will include some of the following.

'Which contraceptive should we use?'

Many girls may worry about whether using the pill will have long-term effects on their health and fertility. Others may have heard about side-effects, but not know enough detail to make a decision. For boys there may be concerns about the type of condom to choose. What is the advantage of one sort over another? Will he look silly if he turns up with the wrong size, or one that has a funny smell? Such questions may seem trivial, but they can feel like matters of life and death to an anxious 16-year-old.

Parents should make sure that young people have the information they need to make sensible decisions. This includes knowing about new contraceptives such as the morning-after pill and the female condom.

'How can I get hold of contraceptives?'

Condoms are very easily obtained nowadays, but getting the pill or a diaphragm may pose more of a problem. Anxiety or embarrassment about making an appointment, or being recognised by someone at the clinic can prevent young people taking that crucial step.

Parents can provide essential support here by offering to accompany a young person to the clinic or doctor.

'Even if I have a contraceptive, how can I make sure we use it?'

This is one of the biggest worries for young people. The negotiation between partners over the use of contraceptives requires self-confidence, maturity and good communications. These characteristics are unlikely to exist for teenagers in the early stages of sexual exploration. To be able to talk about such things with a trusted adult could be of enormous help.

It is difficult for young people to plan their sexual behaviour and to be prepared. It is difficult enough for adults, so it should be no surprise to us to recognise the obstacles faced by young people. It may help parents to look briefly at some of these obstacles.

- Young people may feel that using a contraceptive will spoil the magic moment. The common fear is that stopping to put on a condom or fiddling around with a diaphragm and some jelly will interfere with sex.

- Young people may feel ashamed of planning for sex. They may feel embarrassed or awkward about this, believing that to be seen to have planned for sex will put them in a bad light. This is a particular problem for girls.
- Young people may not know how to get access to contraceptives. This is a point which has already been mentioned. More information about access should be available in schools, youth clubs, etc.
- Young people may have sex infrequently, or it may happen quite unexpectedly. Obviously planning in such circumstances is unlikely. It is precisely because of this possibility that it is worth talking to young people about contraception, even if they are not involved in a steady relationship.

Personal safety

This may be a good place to introduce the topic of personal safety. This probably represents one of the biggest fears that parents have, particularly at the time that their teenagers are first becoming sexually active. Parents have different feelings about boys and girls, and will almost certainly feel more protective and more concerned about the safety of their daughters. This is not always easy to deal with. While some girls may accept, and even welcome their parents' concern, others are resentful that they have to live a more restricted life than their brothers. It is a matter of fact that girls are more vulnerable. For example, they are very much more likely than boys to be raped or assaulted. However, this may not cut much ice with a determined 15-year-old girl, who believes she can handle any situation, and is not keen to be treated like a delicate flower!

Parents need to feel their way in such situations. Being too restrictive can have the effect of increasing tensions within the family. This may lead to conflicts and rows, with the inevitable wear and tear on everyone concerned. In some cases, of course, overprotection may have an effect quite opposite to that intended – the girl may simply refuse to cooperate. The result of this is that parents end up having no influence at all, as their daughter stays out later at night, or stays away for longer periods of time. As with all these things, the best parents can hope to do is to come to an agreement by negotiation.

Let us now look at some of the issues involved in personal safety. First, the effects of drugs and alcohol. This is of course a subject in itself, and suggestions for further reading may be found at the end of the chapter. In the present context it needs to be clearly recognised, by both parents and teenagers, that using drugs and/or alcohol creates additional risk if sexual activity is taking place. It is a sad fact that a high proportion of unplanned teenage pregnancies occur as a result of the girl either having had too much to drink or having used drugs. Using drugs or alcohol impairs judgement. Using these substances makes it that much more difficult for the teenager and his/her sexual partner to be sure that they are properly protected. There is only one conclusion. Sex should only take place with someone you trust, in a setting where you can be *sure* that both of you are safe.

Being out alone at night is another way in which the teenager can be exposed to risk. There are a variety of ways in which parents can help. Don't leave things to chance. Do make sure that your teenagers have a way to get home from a party or late night event. Do make it clear that if something goes wrong, you will find a way of providing help. Do help your teenager plan journeys if he or she is travelling alone and at night. Finally, if your teenager has to pass through places which may be unsafe – certain areas of big cities, for example, or along a lonely country lane – then offer to pay for a taxi, or arrange for some other form of reliable transport. To some this may seem like unnecessary nannying. Nonetheless, parents can play a role where personal safety is concerned. Do make sure you have a thorough discussion on the subject.

> *There's nothing you can do to prevent a physical attack on an innocent young female by some slob of 16 stone. That is why I fear the rape situation. The only preventative measures, if that is possible, is to avoid being in areas where it's most likely to happen – walking alone at night. We've seen on television and the press this last year what happens in railway compartments. Basically you try and encourage your adolescent daughter to be in places where there are people. People tend to form a safety network – a safety net that isn't there when you are on your own.*
>
> *(Father of two daughters)*

In thinking about personal safety we need also to address the issue of assault and rape. A terrible thing like this might happen out of the blue. It may happen simply because someone happens to be at a particular place at a particular time. Nonetheless there are a variety of things that young women can do to make themselves less vulnerable. We have already mentioned two of these: they need to be careful with drink and drugs, and to think ahead if they are going to be out alone at night. We can add others to this list. A young woman:

- should carry a personal alarm
- should consider the possibility of taking a class in self-protection
- should not go out with an older man on her own on a blind date
- should in fact treat all blind dates with great caution
- should not travel alone in the carriage of a train or tube
- should not travel in a car on her own with an unknown man, or group of men. This applies especially after a party, or other similar event

- should be very cautious about the messages she sends if she is out with someone she doesn't know. She should try not to do anything which the man may interpret as an invitation to become sexual or intimate.

It is important for girls, and boys too, to know that there are things people can do in relation to personal safety. Nothing anyone can do will keep them perfectly safe. However all of us can reduce the level of danger to which we are exposed. Sharing this list with your son or daughter will prove a valuable exercise.

Essential messages for parents to emphasise

I want to conclude this chapter by looking at some of the key messages that parents may want to convey in discussions with their teenagers. I have selected a number of points which, in my own experience, seem to reoccur time and time again. Parents cannot hope to be influential in all areas of teenage behaviour. Nor can they expect their children to pay attention to everything that adults consider important. It is for this reason, therefore, that it is worthwhile concentrating on a few central issues, particularly those which are directly relevant to the concerns, questions and anxieties that commonly trouble teenagers.

Sex does not make or break a good relationship

Many young people fear that, unless they are willing to have sex with someone they care about, the relationship will soon end. It is important to talk this through with your teenager. If the relationship between a boy and girl is a good one, then whether to have sex or not is something that can be worked out gradually. If a boy says to a girl that he will only stay with her if she has sex with him, then he is not worth hanging on to.

If you are not sure, say no

This is a point that cannot be emphasised enough. No one should be pressurised into sex. A teenager needs sufficient support from adults so that he or she feels confident enough to resist unwelcome advances.

Contraception is a joint responsibility

Young people, of both genders, should have this message up in large letters on their bedroom wall! The only way a relationship can be genuinely equal is for there to be shared responsibility for contraception, as well as for all other sexual decisions.

Boys should be encouraged to see that they have a role to play in ensuring the personal safety of their partners

They can do this by making sure the girl gets home safely after a date, by not taking advantage of her if she has had something to drink, and, most important, by accepting that 'no' means 'no'. If a girl is unwilling she should not be pressurised into having sex.

Pregnancy and sexually transmitted diseases are a possibility

When you are young it is only too easy to believe that it won't happen to you. The responsibility of adults is to get it across to young people that it can happen to anyone. Sex during adolescence involves risk. No one should be allowed to forget that.

Parents are not obsessed with teenage sex

Young people often feel that their parents are preoccupied with this subject. One girl said in an interview 'My parents don't seem to talk about anything else. They are always asking me "Am I doing it yet?" They may be obsessed with sex, but I'm not'. The

TEENAGERS AND SEXUALITY

problem here is that parents allow their anxieties to show through. These anxieties mean that you do think about the sexuality of your son or daughter a lot, and this comes over as an obsession.

There is also a question of trust involved. Teenagers who sense that their parents are consistently asking questions about their sex life are made to feel that they are not trusted. If at all possible you want to create exactly the opposite impression. The more your teenager feels trusted, the more likely he or she is to share concerns with you.

You will be there, no matter what

Of all the messages that parents need to get across, this one is more important than any other. If teenagers know that whatever happens their parents will be there to support them, then much trouble and strife will be avoided. What do parents want? They want to be loved and respected, they want good communication and they want a continuing influence over their son or daughter. These things are most likely to occur if young people believe:

- that they are valued by their parents
- that they will not be judged too harshly even if they make mistakes
- that they will be supported, even if they get into trouble.

Useful reading

Living with a Teenager by Susie Hayman, Piatkus 1994. Packed with insights and strategies to help understand your teenager's needs. How to negotiate, compromise and foster confidence.

Boys About Boys by Nick Fisher, Pan Books 1993. Written by the advice columnist for a teenage magazine, this frank and informative book covers all the important physical and emotional worries of teenage boys.

Making it: How To Handle Love by Tricia Kreitman, Pan Books 1993. Written by a well-known advice columnist, this introduction to teenage relationships covers first dates, maintaining a relationship, love, sex and contraception.

Teenagers in the Family Produced by the Trust for the Study of Adolescence, this pack, including an audiotape and booklet, covers a range of issues to do with growing up in the family. Available from the Trust for the Study of Adolescence, 23 New Road, Brighton, East Sussex BN1 1WZ. Tel: 01273 693311.

Useful organisations

The Brook Advisory Centre provides contraceptive advice and counselling for teenagers and young people. It is both free and confidential. It also provides advice for parents. For your nearest centre contact Brook at 165 Grays Inn Road, London WC1X 8UD. Tel: 0171 713 9000. There are regional centres around the country.

The Family Planning Association provides a wide variety of services for parents and young people concerned with problems to do with sexuality. They also have a very useful bookshop. Their address is 27–35 Mortimer Street, London W1N 7RJ. Tel: 0171 636 7866.

CHAPTER FIVE

The impact of adolescent sexuality on the family

In this chapter I want to consider how the awakening sexuality of a teenager affects the family. It is probably true to say that, of all adolescent behaviour, early sexuality may pose more challenges for parents that anything else. There are at least two reasons for this. On the one hand, the sexuality of a young person in a family has a subtle but powerful impact on the sexuality of the adults. Adult inhibitions, fears, wishes and needs are inevitably heightened by the fact that a child in the family is taking the first steps towards sexual maturity. On the other hand it is often through sexual expression that the teenager most clearly challenges adult values and adult authority. If parents understand something of what the young person is experiencing at this time, the potential for conflict and difficulty will be lessened. Let us now look at some of the issues involved, including:

- the parents' own sexuality
- boundaries and limits
- sexual activity in the home
- unsuitable relationships
- lone parents
- step-families.

THE IMPACT OF ADOLESCENT SEXUALITY ON THE FAMILY

The parents' own sexuality

I have already mentioned the fact that both children and adolescents are affected by, and learn from the sexual behaviour of their parents. As boys and girls grow and develop, they gradually move closer to solving the puzzle of sex. One element of this search is the child's interest in love. What is love? How do two people love each other? What do two people do together if they do love each other? These are not questions that are usually asked openly by children, but it is not difficult to see how questions such as these may underlie much of the curiosity that is a natural part of growing up.

If we now turn to the issue of how children get answers to these questions, it becomes immediately apparent that children's relationships with their parents are critical here. It is through observing his or her parents that a child first begins to get some clues to these central questions. These clues will be to do with physical contact, with the way the couple talk to each other, with whether they kiss or not, with the fact that they share a bed, with the fact that they want to be alone together sometimes, and so on. The first and most influential model of love must originate from the parents' relationship.

Your child's early questions and concerns will be innocent, in the sense that they may not yet be directly connected to issues of sexual intercourse. However as your child grows up, questions to do with babies, or the facts of life, begin to become important, and so he or she will pay greater attention to your sexuality. We cannot underestimate the importance of the role played by the parents in providing some of the answers to the question 'What is the meaning of sex?'. Of course many other learning experiences contribute. As the young person moves through late childhood and adolescence he or she will be looking outward from the family, seeking answers in the families of friends, neighbours, relatives, and in the media. Nonetheless the sexuality of our parents represents a keystone in the development of each of us.

TEENAGERS AND SEXUALITY

This may seem strange when we think about how young people actually behave in relation to their parents' sexual behaviour. The fact is that young people do find it quite disgusting, indeed revolting, to think about their parents making love. Why should this be so? The strength of feeling should give us a clue. When people feel so strongly about something that they want to shut it out, or deny it, or pretend it doesn't exist, this usually means that it has a powerful meaning for them. It frequently means that quite the opposite is true, that they do want to know about it, or even to be a part of it. This is probably the case here.

All that I have been saying about the importance of the parents' sexual relationship reflects this. To a child it is something so central, so significant, something so connected with envy and jealousy, as well as with the wish to know, that it is almost too much to bear. The teenager defends against this by pushing it away – by saying 'Gross! This is simply too awful to think about'. As one 16-year-old said to her mother, in a well-known TV soap, when told that her mother was pregnant 'God! How horrible! I didn't think you two even did that sort of thing anymore'.

> I know that she's aware about sexual relationships between my husband and me because she has made complaints about being kept awake at night. I remember when she was eleven/twelve when she overheard us making love one night and it really upset her, really really upset her. Actually I haven't talked about this with her for ages but she was absolutely disgusted. She thought that, well first of all she thought that something very unpleasant was happening and she thought that I was in pain and then when she realised that I wasn't she thought that I was absolutely disgusting and in fact she called me a whore and she didn't want to have anything to do with me and, and she couldn't speak to me for a few days. I mean it was really really traumatic for her.
>
> (Mother of two daughters)

THE IMPACT OF ADOLESCENT SEXUALITY ON THE FAMILY

Another important issue here has to do with the parents' own relationship, and how it is affected by the young person's sexuality. I have already referred to this briefly. By the time this happens in the life of a family, the parents may have been together for 15 to 20 years. By this time the passion of the first years will have given way to something quite different. In some cases sex may have ceased altogether, while in others it may be an infrequent Saturday night occurrence. Some couples do maintain a satisfying sex life throughout a long marriage. Research shows, however, that these couples are in the minority.

As a result of this, it may well be that the subject of sexuality is a difficult one within the marriage. If one or other partner feels unfulfilled, and has sexual needs that are not being met, this may cause stress or conflict. Some people find that the waning sexual interest that comes with age is a frightening reminder of physical deterioration. All sorts of emotional issues within the marriage may affect the level of sexual activity between the couple. For example anger or depression are two things which hinder the expression of loving feelings.

All this is of significance because, if sex is a subject surrounded by conflict, then the teenager's sexual activity is going to be that much more difficult to deal with. Without realising it parents may feel jealous or envious of their teenager. It is certainly hard to find that, while your own sex life is virtually non-existent, your son or daughter is having a passionate sexual relationship. Alternatively it may be that parents whose own sexual needs are unfulfilled may seek to experience vicarious gratification through the sex life of their children. There are those who encourage early sexual activity, and enjoy learning about every detail of the teenager's experience. This is understandable, but it is something that parents need to watch carefully.

It is not easy to adjust to the fact that your child has grown up to the extent that he or she is a sexual being. Indeed parents probably have as much difficulty with this idea as teenagers do when thinking about their mother and father making love. All this is relevant, because of the impact it has on the sort of communication that takes place. The hang-ups, the anxieties, the raw feelings that adults have about sex influence the way they talk to their teenage children. To be aware of this is essential if parents are to be able to provide any real assistance and support.

Boundaries

Each family establishes its own boundaries in relation to sexual behaviour. From when the first baby is born the couple gradually establishes how the family deals with things like nudity, sharing the parents' bed, touching the genitals, and so on. These boundaries are significant, in that they are part of the unspoken learning that takes place on matters relating to sexuality.

The family's boundaries come into new focus as the first child reaches puberty. It is at this time that changes need to occur about the way the bathroom is used, about walking around with nothing on, even about the way people touch each other. As a father of two teenage girls I have been surprised at how sensitive I have become about my own body. Once my daughters reached puberty I found that I did not want to be seen naked. Somehow it seemed like an invasion of *their* privacy. I also became very careful about hugs and goodnight kisses. Suddenly I was aware that there were two growing women in the family – not two little girls!

These things will be experienced differently in each family. Nonetheless much of what you have long taken for granted does have to be re-examined as your children enter adolescence. Nudity, for example, now has a quite different meaning. During childhood the fact that members of the family are able to walk around with no clothes on means:

- openness
- trust
- freedom

• a family with no secrets.

Once a boy or girl is a teenager nudity can represent something quite different, something not so positive. It can mean:

• no privacy
• invasiveness
• a lack of freedom.

Parents need to be sensitive to these sorts of things. They also need to be sensitive to the effect of their sexual behaviour on the young person. Just as young people want privacy, they also want their parents to be private too. This becomes especially tricky as far as the parents' sexual activity is concerned.

When children are young, and they go to bed early, the latter part of the evening is a time when parents can be alone. As children grow older, they stay up later. Indeed most families reach a stage when the teenager goes to bed later than the adults. For many couples this may have the effect of reducing their private time to zero. There may not be any time when parents can be confident they will not be interrupted – except perhaps in the early morning. This makes it particularly important that boundaries are respected. Adults can, for example, take care to see that their bedroom door is closed; they can take care to see that the teenager will not have to listen to them having sex, and so on. We expect young people to respect us. They will be more likely to do so if we make it clear that we respect their feelings too.

Sex in the home

How should parents deal with the question of whether to permit teenagers to have sex at home? For many this seems like a really difficult issue – something that leaves you with all sorts of mixed up feelings. Perhaps you want to say no, but can't work out quite why you have such a powerful reaction. Perhaps you want to say yes, but feel that others (your own parents, for example) will be critical of such a decision. It may be helpful to set out the arguments on both sides.

First, let's look at reasons that parents might have for vetoing the idea:

- You will be condoning teenage sex.
- It makes you feel awkward and uncomfortable.
- It could set a bad example to younger brothers or sisters.
- It could leave you open to criticism by neighbours, relatives or close friends.

What about some of the arguments on the other side?

- To say yes implies trust and respect of the young person.
- It acknowledges that the teenager is grown up enough to have a sexual relationship.
- It makes it possible for you, as a parent, to keep in touch with how the relationship is progressing.
- It gives you a chance to get to know your son or daughter's partner.
- It ensures that they will be having sex in a comfortable, protected place, where they will be more likely to use a contraceptive. If they are doing it in the back of a car, or after a party, or out in the countryside, then there is less of a chance that they will have safe sex.

Of course there will be many factors influencing the decision. In the end all families have to weigh up their beliefs and feelings, and take into account all the circumstances. I hope that the list of possible reasons for and against will prove helpful. To my mind it is the final point that tips the balance. As parents we do have responsibilities to assist young people in every possible way to protect themselves against risk. What we want least of all is an unwanted pregnancy, or a case of gonorrhoea. That is the consideration which must, surely, take precedence over all others.

THE IMPACT OF ADOLESCENT SEXUALITY ON THE FAMILY

❝ With my daughter I discovered she was sleeping with her partner in our home. I probably wished it was otherwise, but I suppose being a pragmatist, as it was obviously already happening there didn't really seem much point in saying you'd better go elsewhere. Because I don't know where they would have gone. In the garden, or behind the bus shelter – so I felt uneasy in the early years with my daughter because she wasn't 16 and I suppose there was that whole bit about should I be encouraging it or not. Again I knew there was nothing I could do. She wasn't going to stop once she'd started. Having the boy in the house was difficult. Perhaps I didn't want to have to bump into him the next morning in the kitchen. He used to leave in the early hours of the morning. We all knew what was going on. After it was different because she had a more steady relationship and he did used to stay and he'd be around the next day. It's partly to do with the age with me at which it felt comfortable and OK. After a couple of years with my daughter I breathed a huge sigh of relief and thought "It's alright now, because she's 17 and it feels OK now". ❞
(Mother of two sons and one daughter)

Having said all this, if you do come to a decision that sex in your home is acceptable, the matter should not end there. There are still many issues concerning how your teenager and his or her partner behave. Most important of all is the fact that you – as parents – have probably made compromises in order to come to this decision. It follows that the young people involved should, for their part, show some respect for other members of the family. They too need to make compromises:

• They need to be considerate of younger children.

- They should be sure they don't intrude on others by playing loud music, etc.
- They should not disturb other people's sleep.
- They should be tactful and discreet, and be respectful of the privacy of others. After all they will certainly expect some privacy themselves.

Unsuitable relationships

The problem of teenagers and unsuitable friendships is a broad one, and extends further than the context of this particular book. It is a question which is addressed in 'Teenagers in the Family' and references to this and other books on this subject will be found at the end of the chapter. Where unsuitable sexual relationships occur, many of the same issues present themselves.

The question of what is unsuitable is not an easy one. Parents may consider someone unsuitable for a host of different reasons. At one extreme it may be just that you are not keen on this particular boy or girl. They may be shy or awkward, they may come from a different background, they may have green hair or a tattoo, or they may simply not be 'your type of person'. At the other extreme there may be an objective reason for your concern – they may be using drugs, or may be 15 years older than you son or daughter.

> Well I suppose you just have to find out about it for yourself by doing it. I mean I did, we all did, you've got to make your own mistakes, you can't say to somebody "don't do that because that's gonna hurt you, you're gonna end up really unhappy if you do that". It's unreal, you know you did exactly the same thing and it was the wrong thing to do but you can't live somebody else's life for them by saying "that would be a mistake". Okay you might try to stop someone doing something that would physically

> *hurt them or you know you're not gonna let*
> *someone go off and kill themselves but as far as the*
> *emotions are concerned you've got to go through*
> *it, you just have to.* **'**
>
> (Mother of one daughter)

Parents are faced with an awkward dilemma. If they express their disapproval it is hardly likely to go down well with their teenager. On the other hand to keep quiet and say nothing can be very hard indeed. As in the previous section, I tackle this issue by looking at some of the arguments for and against telling your son or daughter what you think. The reasons for being open and frank are:

- You are being honest.
- To say what you think may make you feel better.
- You believe you are trying to protect your teenager from the hurt that may be caused by an unsuitable relationship.

The reasons against being open and frank are:

- You may force the teenager further into the arms of the unsuitable partner.
- Relationships between you and your teenager may deteriorate as a result of your honesty.
- You may be imposing your standards or your preferences on your teenager.

How can parents deal with this? There are some things which are important to keep in mind.

Parents need to accept that their likes and dislikes may not be the same as the likes and dislikes of their teenager

This may be hard to swallow, but it is a fact of life. You don't expect your teenager to like all your friends. Why should they? They didn't choose them. So, in exactly the same way, there is no compelling reason why you should like the people they are keen on. Allowing young people to grow up and make their own choices in life – in friends and in sexual partners, as in other things – is part of the challenge of being a parent.

Rejecting your son or daughter's lover may be interpreted as a rejection of them too

Young people in early relationships are especially sensitive to how their parents react. They themselves are not sure if they are making the right choice. This may make them defensive. It also makes it difficult for them to hear or take on board any criticism of their partner. Thus a parent who expresses doubts about a teenager's sexual partner will be expressing doubts about the teenager's wisdom and maturity.

What can we conclude from all this? If at all possible parents should go easy on being frank and honest. Teenagers are bound to make some mistakes in their first relationships. These mistakes are essential, as they are part of the learning process. They are the means by which young people sort out –sometimes slowly and painfully – who they want to live with. Parents need to allow some leeway. Someone once said 'Teenagers are apprentice adults'. Part of the apprenticeship is bound to involve making mistakes, and some of the mistakes are going to be sexual ones.

Nonetheless all parents have limits and boundaries, and there will be situations which are intolerable. I mentioned drugs as one of these possibilities. If your son or daughter gets involved with someone who introduces them to the drugs scene, then you will be faced with a cruel dilemma. All the issues raised earlier still apply, but in addition there will be your fears about the effect on your teenager of being encouraged towards the use and abuse of drugs.

Not all families deal with such a situation in the same way. It is worth remembering, however, that you have a right to express concerns about the health and safety of your teenager. In addition teenagers need parents to be open about their values and beliefs. They also need their parents to tell them where the limits are. This may sometimes be counterproductive, leading to a wider rift in the family. More often, however, the young person feels relief that someone has laid down some guidelines. By using these guidelines the young person may find the strength to move back towards safer, less risky and more appropriate behaviour.

Lone parents

Bringing up teenagers on your own is bound to create a range of stresses and difficulties. Some lone parents may have experienced an unhappy divorce or separation. Others may be adjusting to the death of a loved partner. What is certainly true is that lone parents have a range of needs. This is not the place to enter into a lengthy discussion about lone parenthood. Further reading is suggested at the end of the chapter. There are, however, particular issues concerning sexuality which I mention briefly here.

Lone parents can find themselves both lonely and desperately missing the absent partner. As a result of this a parent on their own will almost certainly experience, at some time or other, sadness, depression and a sense of emptiness. Much of this will be emotional, but such feelings are bound to have an effect on sexual need, and may lead to behaviour which affects a teenage son or daughter. It is worthwhile for lone parents to keep in mind the fact that adolescents in the family have needs to. All members of the family may have difficulty adjusting to a complex situation. The following ideas may prove helpful.

Don't compete sexually

The fact that a lone parent becomes sexually available means that he or she may be looking for a partner. This may be exactly what the teenager is doing. It could be therefore that in the same family two generations are struggling with the same issues of dating, making themselves attractive, worrying about their eligibility, and so on. In such situations a sense of competition may be created – the last thing that young people need. After all, for a young person a parent is a source of support and information, as well as someone who can set the limits. If you are a rival to your teenager in the sexual success stakes you will find it that much more difficult to fill the parental role.

Don't flaunt your sexuality

We have already referred to the difficulty young people have in accepting, or even thinking about, their parents as sexual beings. It is not easy, therefore, for young people to be brought face to face with a parent flirting, cuddling, kissing, or showing other signs of being involved in a sexual relationship. Parents should be discreet, if this is at all possible. Your teenager needs privacy, but he or she also needs you to keep some aspects of your life private too. Your sexual behaviour falls squarely into this category.

Maintain appropriate boundaries

This is probably the hardest thing of all for parents to do if they are feeling vulnerable and alone. The teenager will only too easily slip into the role of companion and confidante. This is seductive for the young person, as well as providing much needed emotional nurturance for the adult. Parents should, however, think very carefully about the demands they make on their teenagers in such situations. Where boundaries become blurred the teenager may:

- become over-involved
- obtain too much gratification from meeting the needs of the parent
- be hindered from making appropriate same-age relationships
- feel trapped by the parent's dependence.

THE IMPACT OF ADOLESCENT SEXUALITY ON THE FAMILY

All this is to be avoided. It is always difficult to balance up the differing needs of each member of a family. Adults, however, should keep in mind that they have a role and a responsibility as parents. The role involves keeping some distance and some detachment from the young person. The responsibility involves ensuring that teenagers are free to move gradually away from their parents in order to seek relationships outside the home.

> *Moodiness and temper and, I mean that's always been a problem with us throughout her life. I mean maybe it's a case of being a single parent, it's a very intense relationship. I mean it's always very fraught for most people I'm sure, all other single parents I know have had similar sorts of problems. But she, she was always a very wilful child and so it was sort of tantrums and screams and there were certainly points where I'd have given her away to anyone who would have taken her. We had terrible terrible rows, we used to scream and shout at each other. And you know as she got older there was just an awful lot of this sort of bickering and bitching and sniping at each other. Afterwards I would think you know "why on earth don't I just let it go and ignore it?" I'm drawn into her moods, you know and I always got wound up by it. I didn't really learn how to deal with it properly, I just used to end up time after time sort of sitting in a fume and thinking "Why did I let myself get wound up again?".*
> (Mother of one daughter)

Step-families

There are particular reasons why sexuality in step-families needs attention. The issues surrounding sexuality in step-families are not

74

TEENAGERS AND SEXUALITY

necessarily different from those in other families, but because of the strong emotions and fragility of relationships, sexuality sometimes becomes more overtly important.

We have already noted that all teenagers have some difficulty in accepting their parents' sexuality. Most young people prefer not to think about this subject. In the step-family situation, especially if a parent falls in love and remarries, the children are brought face to face with the parent as a sexually active individual. Young people may find this very hard to cope with. The unusually strong feelings that are created by the sexual behaviour of the parents may lead the teenager to act in a puzzling or strange manner. If you notice odd behaviour ask yourself whether your sexuality has anything to do with it.

Some young people may want to change bedrooms (so as not to be able to hear what goes on at night). Some may avoid outings or activities when the two adults are likely to be together, and others may leave the room abruptly if there is any physical contact between husband and wife. These reactions may appear extreme, but for some teenagers the sexual relationship between parent and step-parent seems at times literally unbearable.

Jealousy is a major issue in all step-families. Clearly jealousy and sexuality are closely linked together. If feelings of jealousy already exist, then evidence of sexuality just makes things worse by emphasising the closeness and intimacy of the man and woman's relationship with each other. It may also be true that an obviously sexual relationship between a parent and a 'stranger' may lead to feelings of jealousy in the teenager, sometimes to a quite unexpected extent.

Another dimension to this subject is the possibility of sexual feelings between adults and teenagers. In intact families, where the parents have seen the children grow up from babyhood onwards, sexual feelings, if they do exist, are usually kept well under control. In step-families, however, the situation may be more difficult because the step-parent may only come to know the teenager once he or she is sexually mature. The possibility that the adult

THE IMPACT OF ADOLESCENT SEXUALITY ON THE FAMILY

will feel sexually attracted to the young person cannot be ignored, and such situations need to be very carefully managed. Where feelings of jealousy already exist, a sense of rivalry may develop between the teenager and his or her natural parent, increasing the likelihood of sexuality being used as a weapon in a family struggle for love and attention.

If a step-parent does feel sexually attracted to a stepdaughter or stepson he or she should not express these feelings, and should not allow them to develop. If at all possible he or she should discuss the matter with the natural parent. If the feelings continue it would be wise to seek professional help. It may be necessary for the two people involved to spend as little time as possible with each other. In some situations the boy or girl may need to live away from home for a while. It is essential to be clear that such feelings must not be allowed to develop.

So far I have discussed the feelings that adults can have towards a stepson or stepdaughter, but the opposite situation can also arise. It may happen that a teenager becomes sexually attracted to a step-parent, and this too can create difficult circumstances. Adults do need to be aware of how they may affect young people. This is especially so at a time of life when teenagers can be impressionable and responsive to the affection of an older person who occupies a significant position in the family.

Many of the things that we have discussed already in this chapter apply as much to step-families as to any other family. However, because of the sensitivities involved, it is especially important for step-parents to maintain the boundaries, and to recognise how easily unmanageable feelings can be created. Here are some guidelines:

- Don't be sexually provocative.
- Don't walk around the house with nothing on.
- Don't dress or undress where you know you can be seen.
- Do keep the bathroom and bedroom door closed. And make it clear to teenagers that you expect the same from them.

- Do maintain your own privacy with your partner. It is not necessary to kiss or cuddle in front of young people. If you are having a passionate sexual relationship do be discreet, and remember the sensibilities of other members of the family.
- Do not intrude on the privacy of the teenager. Privacy is extremely important to young people, especially in a step-family.

Useful reading

The Pill by John Guillebaud, Oxford University Press 1991. This book presents the facts, dispels the myths, and answers the most commonly asked questions about oral contraceptives.

Contraception: A User's Handbook by Anne Szarewsky and John Guillebaud, Oxford University Press 1994. This book provides up-to-date and jargon-free information about the different methods of contraception, including the female condom.

Abortion and Afterwards by Vanessa Davies, Ashgrove Press 1991. This book provides comprehensive information on the medical, legal and practical aspects, from the confirmation of pregnancy, the decision-making process, and the emotional aftermath.

Useful organisations

Parentline offers help and advice to parents on all aspects of bringing up young people. Their helpline number is 01702 559900.

Exploring Parenthood offers advice, information and counselling to parents on issues of family relationships and children's development and behaviour. Their advice line is open from 10.00 am to 4.00 pm Monday to Friday, on 0181 960 1678. You can write to them at Latimer Advice Centre, 194 Fraston Road, London W10 6TT.

The Parents' Advice Centre (Belfast) also offers a variety of services to parents of teenagers. Contact them at Franklin House, 12 Brunswick Street, Belfast BT2 7GE. Tel: 01232 238800.

For general information and advice about step-families contact **The National Step-family Association** Chapel House, 18 Hatton Place, London EC1N 8JH. Tel: 0171 209 2460. Counselling helpline: 0171 209 2464.

Gingerbread is an organisation which provides support, help and social activities for lone parents and their children. They also provide publications. Contact them for your nearest local organisation, at 49 Wellington Street, London WC2E 7BN. Tel: 0171 240 0953.

CHAPTER SIX

Risky behaviour

To take risks often seems to be a natural part of adolescent behaviour. To experiment, to test the boundaries, to sail as close to the wind as possible – all this may appear to be inevitable with teenagers. In fact, as we shall see, there are wide differences between individuals, and many young people remain cautious and conservative. Nonetheless, we do need to understand what factors underlie a teenager's need to engage in risky behaviour if we are to make sense of early sexual development. In this chapter I provide a background by looking at some features of adolescent development, and then move on to explore some of the possible consequences of risk-taking. Issues to be covered in this chapter include:

- the nature of adolescence
- sexual risks
- teenage pregnancy
- sexually transmitted diseases (STDs)
- HIV/AIDS
- assault, rape and exposure to violence
- the parents' response.

The nature of adolescence

As I have already indicated adolescence is best seen as a transitional stage. The young person moves from childhood to adulthood in a slow process. As with all transitions the move from one state to another causes a variety of conflicting emotions. These include:

- anxiety about the future
- frustration at the limitations imposed by adults
- uncertainty about when adulthood has been reached
- loss of childhood certainties
- hopes for success and achievement.

All these concerns lead the teenager to ask some fundamental questions. Let us look at one or two of these.

'When am I grown up?'

Not unnaturally the young person wants to know at what point he or she will be considered to have reached adult status. The problem is that no one can give a clear answer. In our society there are so many different ways of indicating maturity. The law is muddled, and allows people to do some things at 16, some at 17, and some at 18. Parents, teachers, social workers, policemen and so on all have a different perspective on this question. The result of all this is that the teenager often gets frustrated. He may decide to take things into his own hands. She may feel compelled to push the boundaries, challenging adults to say how far she can go.

'What can I do?'

Closely linked to this is the question of what behaviour and what activities are or are not allowed at different ages. This applies to drinking, smoking and staying out late, and it also applies to sexual behaviour. Young people need to know what they can do, and who can blame them? We all need to know what the rules are, and teenagers are no different from the rest of us. (See chapter 8, **Sex and the law**.)

'I want to be different'

Part of the process of growing up involves sorting out who you are. A central theme running through adolescence is 'Who am I?'. To answer this a teenager needs to feel different from his or her parents. A young person can only feel real –an individual, someone who actually exists – if he or she can be sure of being distinct. Being distinct means not being a part of the parent. Psychologists use the phrase 'negative identity' to describe this stage. To paraphrase, the young person is saying 'I don't know who I am, but I do know that I am not going to be like you'. Of course this is only a stage, and teenagers are influenced by their parents and do take on some of their characteristics. For a period in adolescence, however, to be different is essential. It is the only way you can be sure you are you, and not who your parents want you to be.

'Can I do anything at all?'

It is often said that teenagers go through a period when a tiny part of them needs to believe that they are omnipotent – that they can do anything at all. This is closely linked to a belief that nothing can happen to them, that they can handle any situation, that they are all-powerful. Such beliefs are no doubt a defence against exactly the opposite – feelings of intense self-doubt, and fears of not being able to manage anything at all.

All these characteristics of adolescence are associated with the possibility of risk-taking. You want to be grown up, so you need to show that you can do grown-up things. You don't want someone to tell you what to do, so you go over the limit – just to make a point. You have to be different from your parents – they are safe and boring, so you are daring. Lastly you are cool. Nothing can touch you. So why worry about taking precautions?

Sexual risk

When looking specifically at sexual risk-taking it is clear that everything outlined above is directly relevant. There are, however, one or two additional factors which should not be ignored. The first is that freedom can be an intoxicating experience. Some young people may be excessively cautious, wanting to postpone sexual involvement, or wanting to keep it only for a special relationship. However there will be others who may get carried away with the discovery that sex without responsibility is wonderful. Good sexual experiences are very pleasurable indeed. It is not hard to see how in some circumstances teenagers can get carried away with the possibility of unlimited sexual pleasure.

Closely related to this is the fact that some of us are fundamentally greedy. When faced with lots and lots of a good thing – whether it's food, or wine, or sex – there are people who want as much as they can get, and more! Personality factors play a part here, but so does maturity. In order to be sensible, and to recognise that unlimited excess is not always good for us, we need self-control. The ability to exercise self-discipline is something that comes with age, and we should perhaps not judge young people too harshly if this is a lesson they have yet to learn. Parents and other adults can help, as much through example as by anything else. If your teenager sees you grabbing the next cigarette, or the next drink, as if your life depends on it, it will be that much harder for him or her to discover self-control. Parents are role models in so many different ways – even where greed is concerned!

I have already mentioned a common adolescent belief that 'it can't happen to me'. This is absolutely central to the question of whether teenagers are able to avoid risky behaviour. When discussing teenage pregnancy, Professor Frank Furstenberg, an American social scientist, once said 'The issue is not – why does the girl fail to use contraception? The issue is – why would a young person want to take precautions?'. The implication here is

TEENAGERS AND SEXUALITY

that you only take precautions if:

- you are able to plan ahead
- you have a sense of the future
- you have a good reason for not getting pregnant – such as exams, a career, etc.
- you have realised that you are as subject to risk as anyone else.

I believe it is helpful to put the question this way around. In particular it encourages us not to blame teenagers for their risky behaviour. If we can focus on the fact that teenagers need certain characteristics in order to *avoid* risks, we can begin to see just how hard it is for a teenager to be sensible and grown-up all the time.

> *I mean, my friend, she's 14, and as I say you know she lays about with anything and that. And I think it's good we learnt about sex and contraceptives and that early when we did. Because she came from my school. I don't think it's too young because I think we need to know. I think when you get to our age anyway you get, you know, sensual tendencies and you just feel as though you need to. I think even if we hadn't had sex education when we were younger, this would still have happened anyway with her. I think, as I say, at our age you just, you feel that you have to – you have to experiment and that sort of thing. You have to know what life's all about. You only learn from mistakes.*
> *(15-year-old girl)*

Before concluding this section I do need to emphasise that young people vary enormously, and we should be cautious in implying that all teenagers are likely to take risks. As with all things, so much will depend on family circumstances, on the social situation of the young person, and on their individual character. While adolescence may make risk-taking behaviour more likely, this does not mean that all adolescents feel compelled to take risks. Some tread very carefully indeed, avoiding all situations in which there is any danger. Others may tentatively test out their own capacity to cope with risk, but in a limited and cautious manner. Risky behaviour is common in the teenage years. Not all teenagers, however, will be risk-takers.

Teenage pregnancy

It is now time to look at some of the things that can happen as a result of risky behaviour, turning first to teenage pregnancy.

When parents and schools teach about menstruation, and about conception, they rarely give enough attention to the signs of pregnancy. Many girls fear that a late or missed period means that they are pregnant, but of course there can be a variety of reasons to explain irregularities in the menstrual cycle. All girls should know something about this, but they should also know where to go and how to find out if they are pregnant. This is the sort of basic information that no one likes to provide, because to discuss it implies that it might happen.

However it can happen, and it does. Britain currently has the highest rate of teenage pregnancy in Europe, with roughly 9 per 1,000 under-16-year-olds becoming pregnant in 1992. There is nothing more upsetting for a parent of a teenager than to discover that their daughter has become unintentionally pregnant, or that their son is about to become a father. In spite of the possible shock and distress, your reaction at this moment is absolutely critical.

It will have implications not only for how the situation is resolved, but also for the future relationship between you and your teenager. If at all possible stay calm. Don't overreact. If you can support your daughter or son at this stage they will remember it all their lives. It may seem like the end of the world to all of you. If you seek good advice, however, you will come to see that it is not the end of the world, but rather a critical turning point in your teenager's life.

There will be a number of options to consider. If you can consider these with your teenager, so much the better. If you can't, try to make sure that the girl or boy – with his or her partner – thinks through all the possible courses of action very carefully indeed. This is where good advice is worth its weight in gold. The names and addresses of useful organisations are listed at the end of the chapter. Encourage your son or daughter to talk to others, and to take time in making a decision about what to do.

You will have to decide what you as a parent can do to help. Once you are clear about this, do make sure that the teenager understands what assistance you can offer. Parents have a variety of reactions. These may include:

- **Shame**   What will other people think?
- **Guilt**   Where did I go wrong? What could I have done to prevent it happening? Does this mean I have failed as a parent?
- **Anger**   How could my son/daughter do this? He/she has let me down. What a stupid, stupid thing to do!
- **Resentment**   How will this affect me? Will I have a greater financial burden? Will my life have to alter because of the baby?

All these feelings are perfectly normal. An opportunity to air your emotions, and to talk things through with a close friend, a relative, or a professional counsellor will be very important in allowing you to get things in perspective. Do remember, however, that no matter how strongly you feel, your teenager is still a teenager. He or she still needs you. The importance of your support at this point cannot be overestimated.

What are the options? There are essentially three:

- to have an abortion (sometimes called a termination of pregnancy)

- to continue with the pregnancy, and have the baby
- to have the baby, but arrange for it to be adopted at birth.

It needs to be acknowledged that every one of these options has disadvantages. To have a termination may leave the girl with a range of difficult feelings, especially feelings of guilt and loss. Alternatively, the girl may decide she wants to continue with the pregnancy, even though it was unplanned. If so, you need to consider carefully the possible effect on her education and career plans. Questions of childcare, and the future relationship with the father need to be taken into account. Lastly, the baby could be adopted. While some do make this decision, it is not an easy one to see through. All involved should recognise that, once the baby is born, it will be very hard indeed to give it up.

Throughout this section I have talked about the son and daughter, because it is just as possible for a boy as it is for a girl to be in this situation. In thinking about teenage pregnancy there does tend to be very much of an emphasis on the girl and on her situation. She, after all, is the one who will have the termination, or bear the child. Nonetheless the role of the teenage father – or potential father – is one that does need to be highlighted. If there is a strong relationship between the boy and girl it will be that much easier for everyone involved to come to the best decision. Boys too often get pushed to the margins in such situations, preventing them from contributing in the way they would wish. Furthermore, too little attention is paid to the boy's needs for support and assistance. Pregnancy involves two people. There is no doubt that both will be better served if their partnership can be fully recognised by the two families involved.

Sexually transmitted diseases

While everyone has heard of AIDS, not everyone knows that there are many other sexually transmitted diseases. Those most often seen today include gonorrhoea, herpes and chlamydia. Any one of these may well cause far-reaching and distressing results. Although it is important not to frighten people, it is essential that both parents and teenagers are aware of the facts in relation to sexually transmitted diseases (STDs).

- A significant proportion of those who contract STDs are teenagers or young adults.
- The incidence of STDs is higher than it was 20 or 30 years ago.
- Because the pattern and distribution of STDs has changed, and continues to change with alterations in sexual behaviour, there is widespread ignorance about the symptoms of the various common STDs.

For a variety of reasons young people are especially vulnerable to the possibility of contracting an STD. Here are some possible reasons:

- Teenagers may not wish to admit that they are sexually active.
- Teenagers may find it difficult to talk about sex.
- Teenagers may feel invulnerable or omnipotent.
- Teenagers often lack the confidence necessary to obtain information or to seek assistance.
- To take precautions involves planning ahead.

There is a lot parents can do in this area. Talking about STDs is as important as talking about contraception. Don't avoid the subject because you fear being a scaremonger. Be firm ('You must protect yourself'), but also be reassuring ('You can protect yourself').

These are some of the things teenagers must know:

- Anyone who is sexually active can contract an STD.
- The most common way STDs are transmitted is through sexual intercourse.
- AIDS is not the only dangerous STD.

- Many STDs do not have obvious symptoms.
- After abstinence, or only having sex with one trusted person, the best protection against STDs is to use a condom.
- When one person has an STD, so may his or her partner.
- Treatment for STDs is confidential, and widely available (see the end of the chapter).

Anyone who has any of the following symptoms should see a doctor:

- painful burning sensations during urination, or dark coloured urine
- a discharge from the vagina or penis that itches, burns or has a strong odour
- sores, redness or persistent irritation in the genital area
- a persistent sore throat.

When we had a lesson in year 12 about them (STDs) I didn't really sort of think about it at all. I was glad to know about it and then last year I completed a survey at college asking me lots of questions about AIDS and what I knew about it. And I was really quite shocked at how ignorant I was and it wasn't just me, talking to people afterwards, you know, we were all very, very naïve. Although it's always been publicised and we all sort of thought we knew about it, you know questions like, how many people do you think are suffering from it and all this sort of thing. You know, there were things I just hadn't a clue about. I was quite surprised about how little I did know because I thought that I knew a lot more. I think it's made me more careful. A lot more thoughtful about it though. I was just really surprised about what I didn't know basically.

(18-year-old boy)

HIV/AIDS

Because HIV/AIDS has received so much publicity since the mid-1980s, many people believe that they know a lot about the disease. Studies certainly show that teenagers know more about it than about many other aspects of sexuality. Nonetheless there is still much ignorance about the subject. Even among doctors and scientists there are disagreements, both about the causes and about the most effective treatment for HIV infection. In Britain the high level of public anxiety seen in the late 1980s has given way to a different attitude. As figures have shown lower than expected levels of infection among heterosexuals, and among young people, health education campaigns have shifted in their approach, and now focus on groups such as intravenous drug users.

In spite of all this HIV remains the one STD that causes death. It cannot be ignored. Even if rates of infection are low amongst teenagers, that is no reason to avoid the subject, or to stop hammering home the message – AIDS can kill. There are a number of things that as adults we should be certain young people know. These are:

- **AIDS is not a homosexual disease.** Early cases of AIDS did occur primarily in the homosexual community. Today this is no longer the case. Intravenous drug users (whether homosexual or heterosexual) are particularly at risk, as are men and women having heterosexual sex with someone who is HIV positive.
- **There is at present no cure for AIDS.** This may change, but at present AIDS is a disease for which no cure is available.
- **The HIV virus is transmitted through bodily fluids in the male and female sexual organs as well as through blood.** In addition to transmission through sex, an open cut or sore may be a source through which the virus can enter the body.

RISKY BEHAVIOUR

- **Apart from abstinence, the safest protection is to use a condom.**
- **The more sexual partners you have, the greater the risk.**

As with other risk factors, the more parents can inform themselves about HIV/AIDS, the more likely they are to be able to make sure that their son or daughter is well informed. Suggestions for further reading on this topic will be found at the end of this chapter.

Assault and exposure to violence

We have already given some thought to this issue in our discussion of personal safety in Chapter 4. As with all issues like this it is one thing to advise a young person what to do, and it is quite another to see that they take your advice.

In the first place it is important that the teenager, and this applies to both boys and girls, knows that there are things he or she can do to avoid danger. These include:

- recognising that they are not invulnerable. There are circumstances which the young person will not be able to handle
- accepting that there are places, and situations, which are best avoided. These include city areas after dark, being alone in a car with strangers, and so on
- making every attempt to plan ahead. This applies to always having enough money for a phone call or a taxi, to finding out about public transport, and so on.

The possibility of your teenager being exposed to violence is the sort of thing parents worry about when lying awake at 3.00 in the morning. We may fear it yet, strangely, we do not find it easy to talk openly about it. There are a number of inhibitions which prevent us from talking sensibly about the subject of violence.

In the first place even to raise the topic may make you sound fussy and overprotective. It is true that there are teenagers who react badly to expressions of concern about their safety. Nonetheless parents should not be put off by this. You have a right and a responsibility to do everything you can to ensure that your son or daughter remains safe. If your teenager doesn't like it, you need to have a full and frank discussion.

Secondly, you may not wish to raise questions to do with danger and violence, for the same reason that you may be tempted to avoid other tricky issues. To talk about it seems to imply that it might happen. This is simply not a good reason – don't hide behind it.

Third, you may not want to discuss the topic because you don't know what the answer is. We cannot keep our children completely safe. However there are many things we can do. We can:

- make sure that they are well-informed
- let them know that we are concerned about their welfare
- provide them with strategies and options which are available if they need them.

The parents' response

Let us now look more closely at what parents can do. There are in fact two questions to consider here:

- Is there anything parents can do to prevent risky behaviour?
- What should parents do if things go wrong?

Can parents prevent risky behaviour?

The answer to this is probably not. In the end, if young people are determined to drink too much, or drive a car without a licence, or have sex behind the bike shed without using a condom, there is not much parents can do to stop them. However, do remember that not all adolescents are driven to engage in risky behaviour. Many are cautious and conservative in what they do. As for those who do take risks, there are a number of things that can be done which will reduce the teenager's need to challenge adult authority, and so help the teenager to take fewer risks. Here are some suggestions.

- **Keep in mind what it is that your teenager needs from you.** Young people respond best to parents and other adults who are firm but fair. They do not want parents to exercise the heavy hand of authority. That will just cause conflict. Neither do they want a permissive, hands-off approach. They do not want you to say 'Okay, it's your life, get on with it'. This feels like a rejection. Young people need you to steer a middle course – involved and caring, but clear about what you believe in.
- **Show respect.** One of the things young people complain about most is that adults do not respect their point of view. Teenagers do have worthwhile things to say, and they should be given a chance to express their opinions. Often they have sensible suggestions to offer which parents have not even considered. If you are in discussion or in disagreement with your son or daughter, do give them a fair hearing. If you respect them, they are more likely to respect you, and to take seriously your point of view.
- **Be clear about what you consider acceptable.** As I have indicated in previous chapters, young people need to know where they stand. They need to know where the boundaries are. This doesn't mean they will always respect them. They will challenge authority and disobey the rules as a means of defining themselves. Having the rules and boundaries is essential, however, for without them what does your teenager have to hold on to? The boundaries you set create the psychological and internal framework which helps to prevent personal chaos.

- **Be supportive.** Do make it clear that you are there if you are needed. The knowledge that one's parents are available at moments of stress or difficulty is probably the most reassuring thing that teenagers can hope for. However much angst and anger there is, however much shouting and screaming and jumping up and down, teenagers do need their parents. No-one else can take your place. Now, isn't that a comforting thought?!

What should parents do if things go wrong?

However difficult the situation, your response at a time of crisis will have a profound influence on later events. A crisis can happen in many different ways. You may be woken up by a phone call from the police in the middle of the night. You may be called to the headteacher's office. You may discover a syringe under your teenager's bed. A neighbour may tell you something about your teenager which you didn't know. Your son or daughter may, late at night, confide in you a worry about a sexually transmitted disease. All these, and many other things, are possible. What advice is there?

- **If the worst happens, try not to overreact.** However difficult it is, attempt to remain calm. You may feel distressed, furious, ashamed or guilty. Do make every effort to contain your feelings. To paraphrase a well-known saying 'React in haste, repent at leisure'. If you allow your feelings a free rein you may very well regret their effect later on. I know I have said it a number of times already, but remember – in a time of crisis your teenagers need you more than at any other moment.
- **If you do get angry or upset, and you can't contain your emotions, then try to find a way of talking about how you feel.** Be adult yourself. Be honest, acknowledge how strongly you feel, but *make it clear that you are there to help.*

- **Be well-informed.** Whatever the subject, whether it is drugs, STDs or pregnancy, do everything you can to find out about it. Learn as much as you can. This includes seeking out helpful organisations. The better informed you are, the more likely it is that the right decision will be taken.
- **Don't be ashamed to seek help.** Many parents find this the most difficult step to take. To seek help may feel like an admission of failure. It isn't. You will be surprised at how many other families experience similar crises and difficulties. One of the things parents frequently say is that to learn that you are not alone, to find that others are in the same boat can make all the difference in the world.
- **There are some situations where you need professional help.** If you feel out of your depth, or uncertain of what to do next, then ask for advice. You have a responsibility to do so for the sake of your son or daughter. Appropriate organisations are listed throughout this book.

Useful organisations

For advice on pregnancy, abortion and contraception contact **The British Pregnancy Advice Service** at 7 Belgrave Road, London SW1V 1QB. Tel: 0171 828 2584.

Young Minds campaigns to raise public awareness of, and to improve mental health services and resources for, children and young people. They are at 22a Boston Place, London, NW1 6ER. Tel: 0171 724 7672.

The National AIDS Helpline Parents or young people can telephone this confidential helpline. It is open every day, 24 hours a day. Tel: 0800 567123.

The Terrence Higgins Trust Parents or young people can contact this charity for information, advice and help on any aspect of HIV or AIDS. Their address is 52–54 Grays Inn Road, London WC1X 8JU. Tel: 0171 242 1000.

The Suzy Lamplugh Trust This organisation is committed to increasing the personal safety of young people in all ways. It produces videos and other publications, and provides advice and training. The address is 14 East Sheen Avenue, London SW14 8AS. Tel: 0181 392 1839.

CHAPTER SEVEN

Sexual orientation

The process of choosing sexual orientation

It is important to start by acknowledging that all young people, at some time or other, wonder about their sexual orientation. It is an inevitable part of growing up – a perfectly natural question to ask. It is also part of a wider search for an identity which involves the adolescent in trying to work out exactly what sort of person he or she is. There are many components to this search. Some are to do with the sort of relationship the teenager is looking for; short-term or long-term; close, or relatively detached; dependent or independent. Other aspects are to do with plans and goals for the future, while still others concern values and beliefs. In addition to all this, there is the question 'Am I more attracted to people of the same gender as myself or to people of the opposite gender?

This is a question to which there may not be an immediate answer. Although it is true that some people know from childhood or early adolescence that they are definitely gay or straight, the majority resolve this question during the course of their teenage

TEENAGERS AND SEXUALITY

years. Indeed many go through what is known as a transient stage. Thus there are teenagers who have heterosexual relationships but who in due course become gay or lesbian. In the same way there are those who go through a stage of homosexuality – having a crush on someone, engaging in mutual masturbation, or experiencing a full sexual relationship – who become heterosexual adults. What is important to understand is that a period of uncertainty is a perfectly natural part of adolescent development. People do not necessarily have a clear and definite answer to their sexual identity. They may need a number of different experiences, with different sorts of people, before they can be confident about their sexual orientation.

> *I suppose I started having sexual feelings – I didn't categorise them in any way – from the age of 11, I suppose, and those feelings carried on until I was 14, 15. It was only then through watching television, talking to friends, that I would probably categorise some of them, not all of them, as gay thoughts. The actual process of realising that I was one of those 'poof' things that everybody had been talking about at school, was a very long process. It didn't really finish if you like until I was 16, maybe 17, very late on really. I just thought that they were ordinary sexual feelings which in fact they are. It's just that through images and things in the media and social pressures, our sexual feelings get channelled in one direction or the other and in mainstream society one of those sexual feelings is good and okay and normal and the other types are bad and to be got rid of and evil.*
>
> *(20-year-old man)*

In spite of the fact that people know more about homosexuality today, and in spite of considerable changes, both in the law and attitudes, there is still a large amount if ignorance about what it means to be gay or lesbian. Such ignorance has an enormous impact on young people, especially on those who are struggling with queries and uncertainties about their sexual orientation. It is important to emphasise that it is not abnormal to choose a gay or lesbian lifestyle. It is not peculiar or wrong in any way. People who are gay or lesbian are in the minority in our society, but they should not be judged or discriminated against. This needs to be said because, sadly, there is still widespread prejudice against homosexuality.

Prejudice and misunderstanding create a situation in which it is exceptionally difficult for a teenager – indeed for anyone – to be open and honest about the fact that they may be gay or lesbian. Fears about the reactions of friends, teachers and – above all – family mean that most keep quiet. Teenagers in this situation cannot ask for help, and indeed – virtually no support is provided. Young people who are gay or lesbian may thus have to cope with a variety of issues – at school, at work or at home – without being able to obtain the assistance that is normally available to others of the same age.

Finding out that your teenager is gay or lesbian

One of the hardest things for any gay or lesbian young person to do is to tell their parents about their sexual preference. Most teenagers worry for a long time about how and when to discuss the matter. They will almost certainly expect their parents to be upset, or even horrified. All those who are gay or lesbian remember this moment as a very important one in their lives. The reaction of the parents is critical, for it reflects the answer to the question all young people ask: 'Am I still going to be loved and accepted by my family once they know about my sexual orientation?'

TEENAGERS AND SEXUALITY

Why do parents react so strongly? One obvious reason is that parents worry about the prejudice and intolerance that we have already discussed. This prejudice may result in the young person facing difficulties at work, in friendships and so on. Another reason relates to having children. Generally parents want their children to become parents too. This may be:

- because they want to become grandparents
- because they want the family name to continue
- because they have invested so much in parenthood themselves

Of course there are a number of other reasons for worrying about our children's sexual orientation which are less obvious and which involve strong and complicated emotions. Parents want their children to fit in, and to be the same as everyone else. Perhaps most importantly in some primitive way we want our children to be the same as us. All of us have to come to terms with the fact that our son or daughter is an individual. This means that he or she is different – we can't escape this. Deep down, however, we have a sense that our children are a part of us, a part of our identity. Their sexual preference tells us something about their sameness or difference. To find that a teenager is gay or lesbian means that they are as different sexually from a heterosexual parent as they could possibly be.

> When I was 15 I started going to gay pubs and everything which you shouldn't do at that age but it's quite an awful age and I successfully managed to go out for two years until I was 17. It got to a point where I was lying about everything I did, in the family I was lying and I just got fed up with it. So I just came out with it one night. It always comes out like one big thing. When I told my dad he was in bed at the time and I sat on the end of the bed and said "I'm gay". I just watched the colour drain out of

*his face. It was OK to start off with but then he spoke
to my mum and my mum was really upset about it.
I'd sort of led them on letting them think I had a
girlfriend and this and that. That's why they never
had any idea at all. The whole thing sort of erupted
then you know. It was round about Christmas last
year, and it ruined their Christmas anyway, don't
know about mine.*

(19-year-old man)

When parents first find out that their son is gay or that their daughter is lesbian they may well be very distressed. Some may be furious, forbidding the teenager to have anything more to do with homosexual friends. Some may get extremely upset, torturing themselves with guilt about where they went wrong. Others may refuse to discuss the situation, hoping that if they close their eyes, the whole thing may go away. All of these reactions are under-standable, but none will make for good relationships with your son or daughter. Let us look at some of the things parents can do when faced with this situation.

Recognise that this is not the end of the world

It is not easy for parents to adjust to the discovery that their teenager is homosexual. Nonetheless accepting the reality is essential if you are going to be able to continue to communicate with your son or daughter. At first it may seem like a terrible blow. People describe themselves as being 'quite shattered' by the news. However, being gay or lesbian is, as I have said, a choice about our sexual identity. The person is just the same as they were before they told you the news. So remember, this is not the end of the world. Rather, it is the start of a new more honest and open relationship with your child.

Reassure your son or daughter that you still love them

As I have already indicated, the reason that young people have so much difficulty in telling their parents that they are gay or lesbian is that they fear rejection. They fear that their mother and father will turn them out of the home, or refuse to go on supporting them. What young people need in this situation – more than any-thing else – is to know that their parents still accept them, and will continue to care for them. Indeed young people who are gay or lesbian need more support than others, not less. Parents do have a big responsibility here.

> ❛ *Parents should not give an immediate reaction because immediate reactions hurt so much. Because it's taken that child so much courage to actually say something. So just think about what you're saying and go away and think about it. Think about your priorities and if you love that child more than you hate their sexuality. I think you need a lot of time to think.* ❜
>
> *(17-year-old girl)*

One last point. If you feel like rejecting your son or daughter because of their sexual orientation, think again. A serious rift cre-ated at the time you first learn about your son's or daughter's homosexuality will take a long time to heal. In families where this does happen it is all too often the parents who live to regret their actions. The experience of losing a child in this way can be very painful indeed.

Ask to meet your son's or daughter's partner

One clear sign that parents can give to show that they have accepted the sexuality of the young person is to offer to meet the partner. This may not always be appropriate, since obviously in some cases there will not be a steady or serious partner to meet. Nonetheless in situations where your son or daughter is having a relationship with someone who is special to them, then to wel-come this person into your home can seem like a huge step towards acceptance and reconciliation. It may not be easy. You may have all sorts of fears and anxieties. Remind yourself that coming to terms with it all will take time. Meeting your son's or daughter's partner will send a message that you are willing to accept who they are.

> So he sat down and he said "I've got something to tell you and it is important" so I said "alright, what is it?" and he said "well, two of your old friends would understand". And then it suddenly dawned on me which two friends he meant. And it was the gay friends we had. And I just said "oh, so you think you are" and I didn't use the word. And he said yes so I said "well what makes you think that?", he said "I just know". So I said OK, you know that's OK and I could see the relief in his face, and his absolute relief in the whole body. And I just went up to him and he burst into tears. I put my arms round him and said "that's all right, don't worry about it". I said "I still love you, you're my son and nothing's going to make any difference to the way I feel about you. You're no different now than a minute before you told me, so it's all right, don't worry".
>
> (Mother of two boys)

Useful reading

When Your Child Comes Out by Anne Lovell, Sheldon Press 1994. Sympathetic and non-judgmental, this book helps parents come to terms with their feelings when their child tells them they are gay.

Coping With Crushes by Anita Naik, Sheldon Press 1994. This book offers advice and help on how to cope with different types of crushes, on famous people, teachers, girls, boys and people of the same and opposite sex.

Useful organisations

For confidential advice and information about all aspects of homosexuality, contact **The London Gay and Lesbian Switchboard**. They have information on local groups around the country. Parents of gay people are also welcome to phone. Tel: 0171 837 7324.

A helpline is available for parents of gay and lesbian young people through ACCEPTANCE. Tel: 01795 661463. Their address is 64 Holmside Avenue, Halfway Houses, Sheerness, Kent ME12 3EY.

CHAPTER EIGHT

Sex and the law

There are a number of ways in which the laws concerning sexual behaviour affect young people. It is particularly important to consider these laws, since there is widespread ignorance about them among young people. To take an example, a recent survey by the Family Planning Association showed that almost half of teenagers at the age of 15 and 16 did not understand their rights in relation to confidential medical treatment. In this chapter I consider:

- the age of consent
- confidentiality
- sexual abuse.

The age of consent

The law protects children until they are old enough to make their own decisions about sex. The age at which a young person is considered old enough to make these decisions is called the age of consent. If a man or boy has sex with a girl who is below the age of consent this person is committing an offence. In England,

Scotland and Wales the age of consent is 16, although in Northern Ireland it is 17, and in the Republic of Ireland it is 18. In some European countries it has recently been reduced, and it can be as low as 12, as it is now in Holland. This law does not apply to women. A girl or woman cannot be prosecuted for unlawful sexual intercourse if she has sex with a boy of any age, even someone under 16. However there is a possibility that the woman could be prosecuted for indecent assault if the boy was under 16, although such a prosecution is very unusual.

What I have said so far applies to the age of consent for heterosexual relationships. As far as homosexual relationships are concerned the age of consent was 21 until a new law was introduced in 1994. After much debate the homosexual age of consent was lowered to 18 throughout the United Kingdom.

It has to be said that many young people do have sexual relationships when either or both partners are under 16, without realising that they are breaking the law. It is rare for the police to interfere, except in special circumstances. This could be because a parent or guardian objects to the relationship, or it could be that a social worker believes the young person is in 'moral danger'. The grounds of 'moral danger' are sometimes used to take teenagers into care if it is thought they are being promiscuous, or may be involved in prostitution.

Confidentiality

Medical confidentiality is a difficult issue, and one which the law has not found easy to resolve. It should first be noted that anyone of 16 or above has a right to confidential medical treatment. At this age parents no longer have any legal status, in that they cannot insist on being involved or consulted about their son or daughter's treatment.

The difficulty arises if the teenager is under 16. The issue first came to prominence as a result of a court case brought by a Mrs

SEX AND THE LAW

Gillick (a mother of ten) against her local health authority in 1984. She wanted an assurance from the health authority that she would be consulted if a daughter of hers under the age of 16 sought contraceptive advice. The health authority refused to give such an assurance, and in the end the case went all the way to the House of Lords.

The Law Lords ruled against Mrs Gillick. They argued that, in certain circumstances, someone under the age of 16 should have the right to confidential medical treatment. The conditions they attached to this right were as follows:

- that the girl (although under 16 years of age) will understand the doctors advice
- that the doctor cannot persuade her to inform her parents or to allow him/her to inform the parents that she is seeking contraceptive advice
- that the girl is very likely to begin or to continue having sexual intercourse with or without contraceptive treatment
- that unless she receives contraceptive advice or treatment her physical or mental health or both are likely to suffer
- that her best interests require the doctor to give her contraceptive advice, treatment or both without parental consent.

Lord Fraser, in considering the question of parental rights, made the following statement:

Parental rights to control the child existed not for the benefit of the parent but for the child. It was contrary to the ordinary experience of mankind, at least in Western Europe in the present century, to say that a child remained in fact under the complete control of his parents until he attained the definite age of majority, and that on attaining that age he suddenly acquired independence.

In practice most wise parents relaxed their control gradually as their child developed and encouraged him to become

TEENAGERS AND SEXUALITY

increasingly independent. Moreover, the degree of parental control actually exercised over a particular child did in fact vary considerably according to his understanding and intelligence.

It would be unrealistic for the courts not to recognise these facts. Social customs changed, and the law altered and did in fact have regard to such changes when they were of such major importance.'

I quote this in full because it is an important statement. Apart from Lord Fraser's use of the word 'he' when he is talking as much about girls as boys, the statement represents a recognition of the changing nature of adolescence, and of the gradual shift in parenting behaviour that is so essential as teenagers mature.

Since the Gillick judgement, the Department of Health, as well as numerous public health bodies, have sought to clarify under exactly what conditions young people can expect confidential treatment. There has unfortunately been much confusion, with the result that many teenagers – and indeed many adults – are unclear exactly what the situation is. To summarise:

- No doctor can be prosecuted for aiding and abetting unlawful sexual intercourse if he or she provides contraceptive advice to someone under 16.
- If a teenager under 16 asks for his or her parents not to be informed, a doctor has to make a personal decision as to whether that individual has reasonable grounds for seeking confidential treatment.
- In practice doctors vary in the position they take. As a result it is difficult for a young person to be sure if they will or will not receive confidential treatment.
- Very few GP surgeries provide family planning services for young people which are truly user-friendly. Most do not fully take into account the needs of young people.
- In almost all towns and cities there are advice and

information services for young people which do guarantee confidentiality. Brook clinics are a good example of such a facility. However young people who live in rural areas are disadvantaged, since access to such services is more difficult.

Sexual abuse

This is the sort of subject no one likes to think about. Yet we know that large numbers of children and young people are sexually abused each year. All parents should be aware of the problem, and should learn something about the circumstances surrounding sexual abuse. This is especially true if the adult is also a teacher or youth worker, or is someone who comes into contact with young people in their work.

It is important not to oversimplify, since every individual circumstance will be different, and any guidelines there are can only be of the most general sort. It needs to be absolutely clear, however, that:

- incest – a sexual relationship with a close relative – is a criminal act against the child or young person
- sexual assault is also a criminal act against the child or young person
- sexual intercourse or any other kind of sexual intimacy by an adult with someone under 16 is an offence against the young person and can lead to prosecution.

Sometimes it is hard for adults to believe that someone they know has been sexually abusing a young person. This can mean that the honesty of the child or teenager is doubted by those around them. If you are in this situation, remember it is not easy to make up a story about sexual abuse. It is highly likely that what you are hearing is the truth.

It is often believed that so long as the actual abuse can be prevented from occurring again, the whole matter is best forgotten. Sadly this is not the case, since adults who sexually abuse young people may be unable to stop, and may well go on to abuse other children in the family, or others whom they know well. Also, the young person who has been abused will need help to undo the damaging effects of the abuse once it has ended.

If you suspect that a child or young person you know is being sexually abused, you have a responsibility to talk about it – however awkward or disagreeable that may be. Do seek professional help. If something can be done you will be protecting not just the young person you know, but possibly many others as well.

If, as an adult, you are sexually abusing a young person you must seek help to stop this happening. Many adults who do have sexual relationships with children tell themselves that it is all right, because the feelings they have are loving feelings, not simply violent ones. This is far from the truth. For a child or a young person to be forced to have sex with a trusted adult is one of the most damaging experiences possible, whatever the feelings of the adult may be.

Some adults say that their instincts tell them it is wrong, but that they do not have the strength to stop themselves. Also, adults can easily convince themselves that the young person doesn't mind, or isn't being affected by the experience.

If you are in this situation seek help now. Do not allow your sexual feelings towards the young person to be expressed openly. If they are being expressed, find a way to stop yourself. You may feel ashamed, or afraid of telling someone. It may well be difficult for you, but if you do have loving feelings towards your child or teenager then you will want to prevent them from being damaged any further.

Useful Organisations

The Children's Legal Centre. *This organisation can be contacted for advice about any legal matter to do with children or young people. Their address is PO Box 3314, London N1 2WA. Tel: 0171 359 9392. Advice Line: 0171 359 6251.*

Citizens Advice Bureau (CAB). Trained CAB workers offer information and advice on a wide range of topics, including legal problems and family and personal difficulties. Anyone can use the CAB, but you may need to make an appointment, or you may be able to call in and wait your turn. Some CABs give advice over the telephone, but lines tend to be very busy. To find your nearest CAB look in the telephone book under "Citizens", or ask at your local library.

CHAPTER NINE

The parents' role

In this final chapter I look at some of the issues facing parents as they come to terms with the sexuality of their son or daughter. The topics I cover include:

- the generation gap
- managing conflict between parents
- communication
- recognising problems
- coming to terms with adolescent sexuality.

The generation gap

The phrase 'the generation gap' is sometime used to refer to a difference in values or attitudes between two generations – particularly between teenagers and their parents. It is a phrase frequently used by the media. It is also one that all too easily becomes linked with sensational or frightening ideas, such as 'generations at war' or some similar notion.

In fact research shows that parents and teenagers do have differ-

THE PARENTS' ROLE

ent opinions on some subjects, but not on all. There may be differences about sex, but not about honesty, or politics. Furthermore, having a difference of opinion does not necessarily mean being in conflict, or being at loggerheads. It is possible to agree to differ.

Research also shows that families vary enormously in the extent to which the generations agree or disagree on sexual matters. Parents of young people are more likely to share values, and to have similar opinions about sex, when communication in the family is good. The more discussion there is, and the more respect the generations show for each other, the less the chance of conflict.

Nonetheless sex is a matter on which parents and teenagers may well disagree. This is not really surprising, if we think of the enormous changes that have occurred over the last 40 years where sexual behaviour is concerned. The dramatic changes in society – caused, for example, by the availability of the pill, the women's movement, changes in censorship laws, and the existence of HIV/AIDS – have meant that the experiences of one generation are bound to be quite different from the experiences of another. Thus we cannot really expect people born 30 years apart to have the same values in relation to sexuality.

> ❛ I think there is a generation gap full stop. I know even with our youngest son, I can't quite remember what the context was, but he turned round to me and said "you're so Victorian". I'd hate to think I was Victorian. I think attitudes to things like sex change so violently even in a space of 10 to 15 years, parents aren't always going to be able to keep up with the way the younger generation are thinking on these things. ❜
>
> *(Father of three sons)*

Particular difficulties arise for young people growing up in minority ethnic cultures. Thus it may well be that a Moslem girl, for example, finds herself torn between two sets of cultural standards, as well as between two generations. Parents who are Asian, or Turkish, or

African, may face the problem of ensuring that their values – often rooted in their own religious background – are upheld. Yet they and their children may live in a society in which quite different values are dominant. Differences between cultures may widen the gap between teenagers and parents in such circumstances. Parents need to recognise that the importance of maintaining their cultural values – especially where sexual behaviour is concerned – may create particular strains for their sons and daughters.

If you find that you disagree with your teenager about sex, try not to let it become a major barrier between you. Remember:

- young people are entitled to hold different views
- young people are *likely* to hold different views, given their different experiences
- people with different views do not necessarily need to fall out
- communication is still possible, even if the other person has an opinion which is different from your own!

Managing conflict between parents

I have talked a lot in this book about the possibility of disagreement between children and parents. However, no attention has yet been paid to another sort of conflict within the family – that between the parents themselves. Of course all couples differ in the extent to which they come into conflict with each other. Some couples hate arguments, and manage disagreement by allowing one partner to dominate. Others avoid conflict by each going their own way. In some families there may be battles and arguments over the smallest things, while in others there may be complete harmony.

Most couples find one way or another of sorting out between

THE PARENTS' ROLE

them how they will manage their children. Of especial importance here is managing issues which can cause friction. Parents learn that it is best to show a united front. If children can drive a wedge between parents, playing one off against the other, relationships in the home are likely to deteriorate. It is not good for children to have the power to create disagreement between their parents.

Many parents find, however, that the relationship comes under strain when there are teenagers in the house. The sorts of issues we have been discussing – challenging behaviour, testing the boundaries and so on – do push parents to their limits. To their distress parents find that as a result of this they are rowing or disagreeing with their partner in a quite unexpected manner. This is especially difficult, since it may be just at this time that parents most need each other's support.

There are some teenagers who have the capacity, not just to wind adults up, but to create tensions between their parents too. If this is happening in your family try to step back and look closely at what is going on.

- Have rows between you and your partner increased as a result of your teenager's behaviour?
- If so, ask yourself what the arguments are about.
- Try to see the situation from the perspective of an outsider. You may realise how much you are being affected by the teenager's behaviour.
- If necessary, talk to a trusted friend. This may help you to see things in a different light.
- Find a way to talk to your partner quietly and calmly, preferably away from home. An evening out or a short holiday may be a good time to do this.
- Your teenager may be getting a buzz from seeing you at sixes and sevens. Don't let this happen.
- Remind yourself that your teenager needs his or her parents to be in agreement, not in conflict.

Communication

I have referred a number of times throughout this book to the importance of communication. Yet communication on the topic of sexuality remains a difficult area for parents, so let us look in this final chapter at some of the obstacles, and consider what can be done.

Obstacle 1: 'I am too embarrassed to talk about this'

Many people do feel embarrassed. You are not unusual. Why not start by letting your teenager know that you think it's important to talk, but that you feel embarrassed to do so? To acknowledge this may be helpful to both of you, and bring you close enough together to start the process of sharing your views.

Obstacle 2: 'My teenager won't tell me what he/she is doing'

Many parents gets discouraged or upset because they feel their teenager is not being open and honest about their emotional life. Parents should not expect teenagers to do this. Because of their uncertainties and anxieties young people need privacy as far as their relationships are concerned. Communication about sexuality – about contraceptives, sexually transmitted diseases, and so on – is not the same as sharing every intimate detail.

Obstacle 3: 'I want to talk, but my teenager avoids the subject'

This situation occurs most often because the subject is tackled in the wrong way. Don't force the issue. Choose a moment when your teenager wants to talk. Start by letting them set the agenda. Use a TV programme or another event to open a discussion. Above all, show that you are willing to listen. A good listener is the best communicator.

Obstacle 4: 'I am worried that if we do talk about sex, we will end up in violent disagreement'

This is another common worry. You may find that you and your teenager disagree, but does this have to mean a violent row? Try to accept each other's differences. If you can do this you will be accepting that your son or daughter is an individual in their own right.

Obstacle 5: 'I feel completely out of my depth. My teenager probably knows so much more than I do'

There are two ways parents can tackle this. First, they can make sure they are well-informed by reading up on the subject, or by watching a video. Your local library will help you. Second, you can be honest with your teenager. If you tell your son or daughter that you are worried about your lack of knowledge, you may find he or she will be much more open too. Having a good discussion may reveal that you have both got things to learn from each other.

> Well I'd say no matter how hard it is, grit your teeth, giggle and get it out. Get it out of your mouth because once you've got it out the first few times it is easier. All I can say really is take a deep breath and have a go. Speaking about it, talking about it. And if you say, I don't know, "I got this book out of the library because I realised that I didn't know that much and I thought we could learn this together" or whatever, I don't know, but take a deep breath and go for it.
>
> *(Mother of two sons)*

Communication about sex may seem difficult or even impossible to some parents. However, communication is a skill that everyone can learn. You do not have to be clever with words, or have passed lots of exams, to communicate well. Some of the most powerful communication occurs between people without any talking at all. If you want to get through to your teenager, there is a way to do so. The suggestions I have made will, I hope, prove helpful.

Recognising problems

Some parents may be faced with adolescent behaviour which they do not understand. Others may worry that something the teenager is doing is abnormal, and requires treatment or professional help. For example you may come home one evening and find your son watching a pornographic video. Alternatively your daughter may seem to be promiscuous in her sexual relationships. She may be sleeping with a different boy each week, and be proud of it. Perhaps you find girls' clothes in your son's bedroom, and you worry about cross-dressing, or some other unusual behaviour. What do parents do in such circumstances?

This is not the place to discuss problem behaviour in any great detail. Indeed each problem will probably be unique in its own way. The difficulty for parents is to know whether a particular behaviour represents an illness or disturbance, or whether it is within what we might call 'normal limits'. Another problem here is that even if the parents believe the young person's behaviour to be serious enough to require treatment, the boy or girl may not take the same view.

The first thing to say is that if parents are worried, they should seek professional advice. You may not need to involve your teenager at this stage. An initial discussion with your GP, for example, may reassure you that no further action is needed. Such a consultation may be enough to allow you to see the behaviour in a different light. You may learn that something you are worried about happens quite often, and that your teenager's behaviour is perfectly normal.

Of course this first meeting with a professional may have quite a different outcome. It may be that your teenager's behaviour does need some attention. The doctor may persuade you that your teenager does need help. You are then faced with the question of how to involve your son or daughter. However difficult it is, you need to clarify with them what they feel about the behaviour. Are they worried? Do they feel that counselling, or some other form of treatment would be helpful? It may be very tricky indeed to discuss this. You will need patience and sensitivity. If you as parents are worried, however, you can share this concern with your son or daughter. Try not to be critical, or domineering. If you express your concern in terms of an anxiety about the welfare of your child you may find it possible to talk about it.

You need to be prepared for a number of different reactions. Your teenager may be defensive, and deny that there is a problem. They may be angry and resentful that you have interfered. However, many young people will be relieved and grateful. All too often adolescents struggle with a deep-seated fear about their strange or eccentric behaviour. They are unable to seek help themselves, but need someone else to acknowledge that they may have a problem. If parents can do this for their son or daughter, they will have done something very important indeed.

Coming to terms with adolescent sexuality

It is no easy task for parents to come to terms with their son's or daughter's sexuality. I have referred to this issue a number of times in the course of this book. When a young person starts having a sexual relationship this is symbolic of maturity. It represents, more clearly than anything else, the fact that the child is now grown up. Of course one of the dilemmas of today's world is that the 14- or 15-year-old who is sexually active may appear to the parents to be

TEENAGERS AND SEXUALITY

far from grown up. Nonetheless sexuality is connected with adulthood. It is also connected with identity and individuality. The teenager who is sexually mature is an individual. He or she is someone who has an intimate relationship with a partner outside the family. He or she is someone whose actions state 'I am now a separate person'.

Mothers and fathers have to make a considerable adjustment in order to accept this change in status. Their child is no longer a child. In order to come to terms with this adults have to let go, and for some this may be very hard indeed.

To conclude this book I shall turn to three parents – two mothers and a father. What they have to say underlines the advice I have been giving. Their experience will, I hope, prove helpful to all parents struggling with teenage sexuality.

- Accept, but don't always approve.

> I feel that no matter how much you disapprove of the youngster's sexual attitudes the chances are they're gonna do it anyway, and you have to decide whether you are going to bridge the gap and try to understand what they do or risk them just deceiving you. So you may just have to look away and accept what you don't approve of. And there is a fine line between acceptance and approval.

- Play the listening game.

> A parent plays the part of a shoulder to cry on, support, the knowledge base. It's almost like a waiting role or a listening game but being aware, and showing the child that you are available for anything, even if it's relatively trivial.'

- Be willing to cut the cord.

> There comes a time when we have to let our children go their own way. We have to cut the cord

THE PARENTS' ROLE

and we have to take them by the hand and say "Go and get on with it". We can't do it for them once they've flown the nest, or once they've become sexually active. We cannot take them and give them a condom to wear and say "Here you are, you've got to use it". It's up to them.

Good luck.

Index